My goal as a yoga instructor is to raise our capacity to live a more vital, compassionate, engaging and meaningful life. Knowledge of the chakras supports a greater awarness in the practice of yoga and in our lives. Sandra and I are interested in showing a more energetic view of the chakras than is commonly seen. We hope this book will enable you to tune in to all the 'energy channels' we have available. The chakras can be a point of entry into increased awareness, enabling us to listen and respond to our experiences with heightened vitality – actually enhancing communication between our brain and body. The unique combination of movement, meditation, breath and affirmation balances energy. It increases blood flow, and can even promote beneficial physiological changes in the brain.

My goal as a yoga instructor is to raise our capacity to live a more vital, compassionate, engaging and meaningful life. Knowledge of the chakras supports a greater awarness in the practice of yoga and in our lives.

Artistic expression helps us see and feel things more powerfully

It is important to me to include the art of my dear friend, Sylvia Hamilton Goulden. She helps us 'see' and 'feel' things more clearly by highlighting human energy through her use of line, shape and color.

SUSAN

The work of Dr. Candace Pert, the renowned neuroscientist, and author of *The Molecules of Emotion*, was my first introduction to 'Mind Body Medicine.' Her large body of scientific research demonstrated the connection between emotion and biology. By showing that serotonin (a compound which modulates mood) is largely produced in the intestine, she validated the biology behind 'gut instinct.'

This area - the lower abdomen - corresponds both anatomically and energetically to the solar plexus chakra. When something bad, sad or frightening happens, a foreboding feeling is typically experienced in the abdomen due to the outpouring of serotonin there, and not in the brain as was traditionally thought.

Deepak Chopra, the prominent alternative medicine advocate, public speaker and writer, has acknowledged that much of his work was made possible through Candice Pert's original research.

In her article, **"Hardwired for Bliss,"** Candice states: *"Another obstacle to experiencing pleasure today may be the thought that we are separate from each other and from the rest of creation. We really are all one. When you start to get this, maybe even only on a subconscious level, I think you will start to experience more bliss."*

SUSAN & SANDRA

For many years we have independently been influenced by the work of Louise Hay on the healing benefits of positive thinking. Her work has inspired us. By connecting positive affirmations to each chakra, we fortify our intention and focus our energy. This is our version of emotional detox.

"When we are ready to make positive changes in our lives, we attract whatever we need to help us."

"Every thought we think is creating our future."

"Peace begins with me. The more peaceful I am inside, the more peace I have to share with others."

"My intuition is always on my side."

"All that I need to know at any given moment is always revealed to me."

"The point of power is always in the present moment."

"I will not be distracted by noise, chatter or setbacks.

Patience, commitment, grace will guide me."

These seven quotes... Louise Hay

"I will always have enough. I will always be enough."

Susan Cambigue Tracey

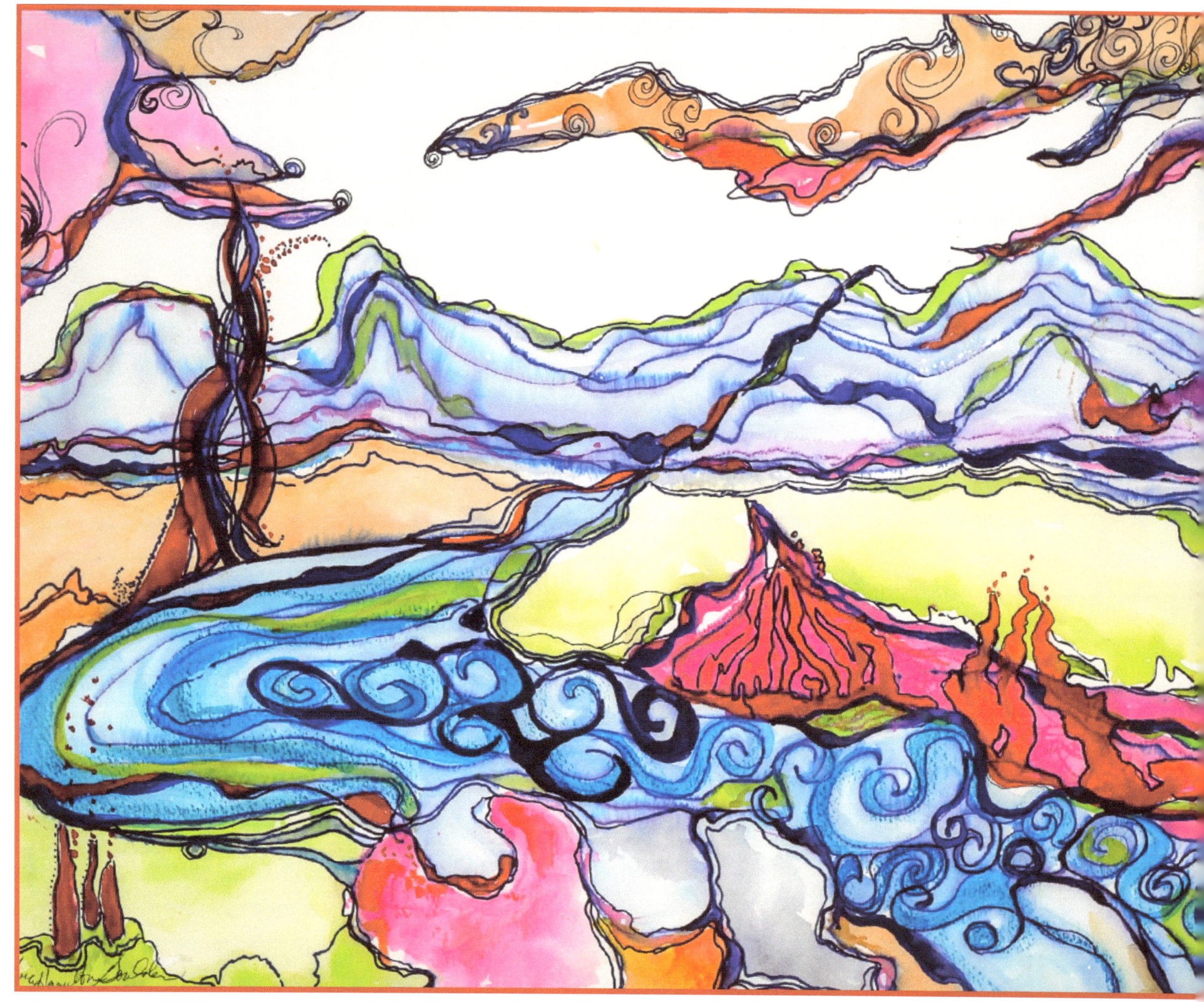

AN INTRODUCTION TO THE SEVEN CHAKRAS

Sanskrit is the primary, sacred language of Hinduism and is a central, foundational component in Inda-European culture and studies. The term chakra means 'wheel' in Sanskrit. In the context of the Seven Chakras, the term refers to the wheels of energy along the spine, beginning at the region centered on the tailbone and continuing upward through the crown of the head and above.

In Hindu philosophy, the chakras are grouped into three areas: the lower chakras (Root, Sacral, Solar Plexus), the middle chakra (Heart), and the three upper chakras (Throat, Third Eye and Crown). These last three are best awakened and balanced through meditation. Together, these seven energy wheels are a fundamental component in the study of yoga.

According to the Bhagavad Gita, one of the most sacred of Hindu texts, the chakras are believed to be part of the 'subtle body,' which is comprised of the mind, intelligence and ego.

Each chakra is associated with a specific location in the body, a particular color, and has an emotional and physical impact on its related organs and glands.

We have provided suggestions for affirmations (mantras) which can be used to strengthen a specific chakra. Finally, we will share a simple sequence of hand gestures (mudras) combined with basic breathing techniques (pranayama).

Breathing with awareness (Pranayama)

Breath helps us move energy throughout the body. The benefits of a regular daily practice of simple, deep breathing include:
- Focusing the mind and attention
- Reducing anxiety, anger and depression
- Lowering/stabilizing blood pressure
- Increasing energy levels and vitality
- Integrating all body systems
- Relaxing physically, mentally and emotionally
- Decreasing feelings of stress - being in the moment
- Balancing the Autonomic Nervous System

"The heart and the lungs are the mother and father of the body."

Susan Cambigue Tracey

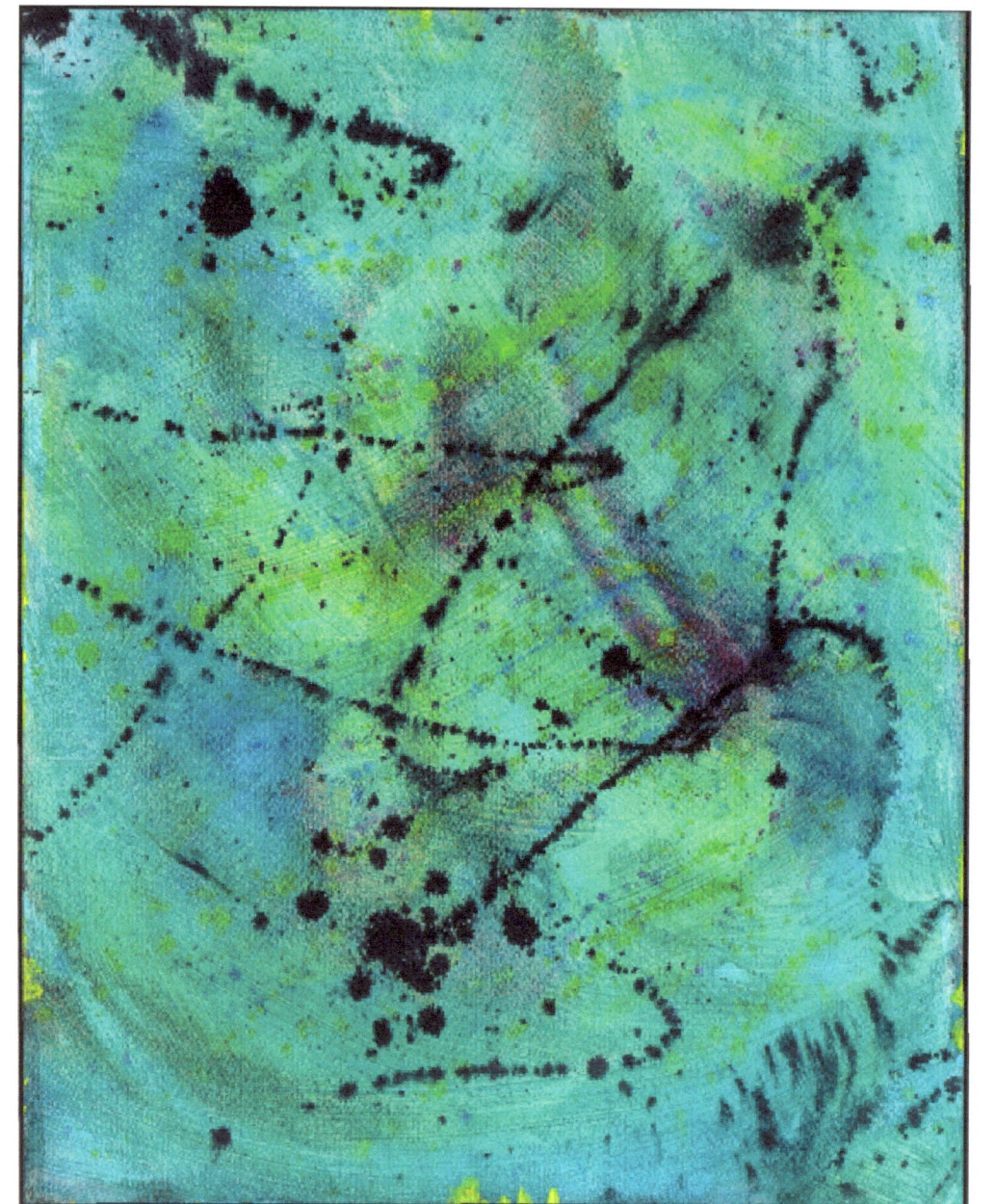

SANDRA

We created this moving meditation to synchronize the breath with the seven chakras. With the addition of affirmations, we can harness our personal power to develop our life's vision by literally rewiring our brain.

The ANS operates through an immense neural network which innervates the organs of the chest, abdomen and pelvis. It courses through the spinal cord and in large nerves, including the Vagus Nerve which is responsible for the relaxation response.

Contraction of the diaphragm produced during inhalation (the breath) activates the Vagus Nerve. Hence, conscious breathing brings us in direct contact with our sensory experience. As such, the breath is the only part of the ANS which is consciously

The breath is much more than the input of controllable. We can harness the breath to oxygen and the removal of carbon dioxide. It manage unresolved emotion (stress) which can connects us directly to a part of the nervous have a 'wind-up' effect on the Autonomic system called the Nervous System. This can then be modified by Autonomic Nervous System (ANS). The ANS breathing ourselves 'down,' making it possible to balance our energy.

SUSAN

There are many different ways of working with the breath. We have provided three choices.

1. **Pranayama:** *Four count breathing with pauses.* Inhale through the nose for 4 counts - pause; exhale through the nose for 4 counts - pause.

2. **Pranayama:** *Ujjayi or diaphragmatic breathing,* also known as 'Ocean Breath' because of the sound produced. It activates the muscles of the lower abdomen (first and second chakra), the rib cage (third and fourth chakras) before moving into the upper chest and throat (fifth chakra).

Inhalation and exhalation are done through the nose and should be equal in duration. The length and speed of the breath is controlled by the diaphragm which is itself strengthened by Ujjayi.

3. **Pranayama:** *Mouth/nose breathing variation.* Inhale through the nose - pause; exhale through the mouth - pause; inhale through the mouth - pause; exhale through the nose - pause.

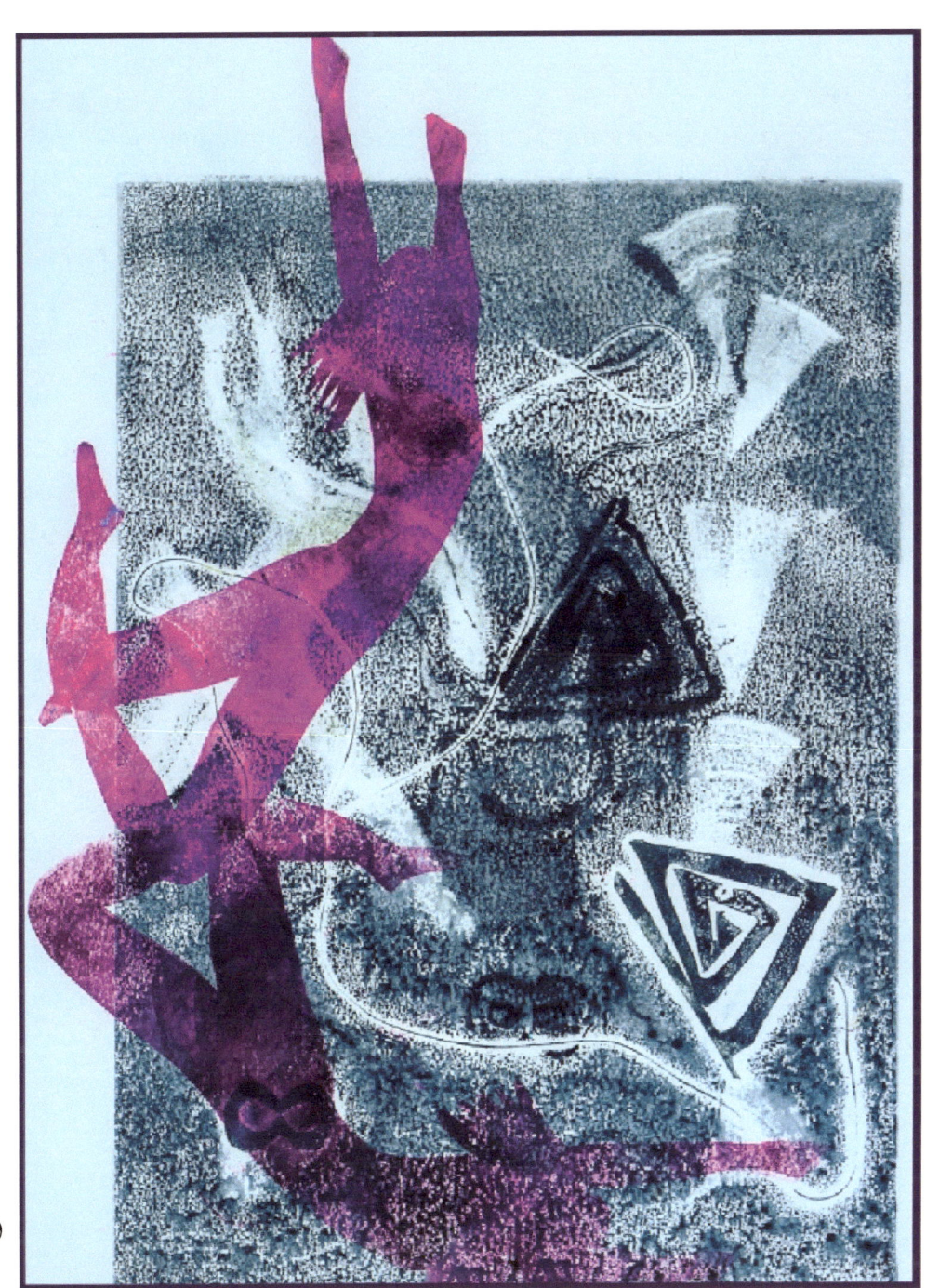

SANDRA

We are emotional beings. Science is now beginning to understand how emotion affects us neurologically. In response to emotion, physical changes in the brain can be mapped using a technology called functional MRI or fMRI. A study published by Carnegie Mellon University investigated the response of the brain to emotion. By using fMRI, investigators were able to identify areas of the brain associated with specific emotions. Each emotion produced a distinct neurological signature. The process by which brain cells do this is called neuroplasticity, derived from the root words 'neuron' (meaning brain cell) and 'plasticity' for the capacity to be sculpted or molded.

Accordingly, the brain has the potential to create new neural pathways to reset or reorganize itself, depending on how it has been used or not used. Like a muscle, areas of the brain become larger or stronger the more they are used.

Conversely, unused areas become weaker and atrophy. For example, every time we experience being 'stressed out' the areas of the brain responsible for this specific response are reinforced and grow stronger. Meantime, the neural pathways responsible for being 'calm, cool and collected' are neglected and grow weaker.

This concept of *Neurons that fire together, wire together* was described by Donald Hebb, a Canadian neuropsychologist. Our ha-bitual thoughts, feelings and behavior actually fortify neu-ral networks. There is evidence that the birth of new brain cells (neurogenesis) can occur in adults and even persist into old age. Unlike old dogs, you *can* teach an old brain new tricks!

Meditation is a most powerful tool which can be used to harness the brain's ability to reset itself Studies have linked the practice of meditation to increases in the volume and density of grey matter (neuroplasticity). At the University of Wisconsin, scientist Richard Davidson, in association with the Dalai Lama, studied the effects of meditation on the brain. His results indicate that meditation promotes neurogenesis in areas of the brain associated with emotion and executive function.

You don't have to be a Tibetan monk to create new neural pathways. Dr. Sara Lazar, Harvard Medical School, has demonstrated that meditation produces changes in brain structure in as little as eight weeks.

We also know that the areas of the brain associated with cognitive function (thinking, reasoning, evaluating, judging, remembering) are also activated by movement. So, whatever you think, perceive and feel (consciously or not) while you are in motion, essentially trains the brain to think, perceive and feel more. Mind and body align. Our attitude, judgments and self dialogue are every bit as important as the breath when we practice yoga.

Our brains are proving to be more flexible than we ever thought possible. This is why it is of critical importance to pay attention to the ways in which we speak to ourselves. Are we kind in our self assessment? Would we speak to others the way we speak to ourselves? Would we let others speak to us in the same way? Our individual thoughts and associated emotions determine the structure of our neural pathways and, as such, are essential in laying down the architecture of our lives. So, how you use your mind changes your brain – for better or worse.

Your beliefs become your thoughts,
Your thoughts become your words,
Your words become your actions,
Your actions become your habits,
Your habits become your values,
Your values become your destiny
Mahatma Gandhi

Affirmations are a method by which we can rewire negativity. The brain re-patterns itself based on both positive and negative thoughts and emotions. This is particularly important because the human brain has a natural tendency to hold onto negative experiences over positive ones. A repeated, positive thought speeds up neuroplasticity

Affirmations should be crafted to reflect goals and repeated often, especially during periods of meditation and relaxation. They can be altered as goals change or are achieved. When choosing an affirmation, it is optimal to use the correct language. Say: *"I am becoming,"* rather than *"I am."* For example, if a person says, *"I love myself,"* and repeats it 10,000 times daily, the brain will sarcastically counter every single time with, *"Really? Sure you do!,"* defeating the affirmation. If the person says, *"I am becoming more loving to myself,"* the brain is disarmed. Positive neural pathways will ensue.

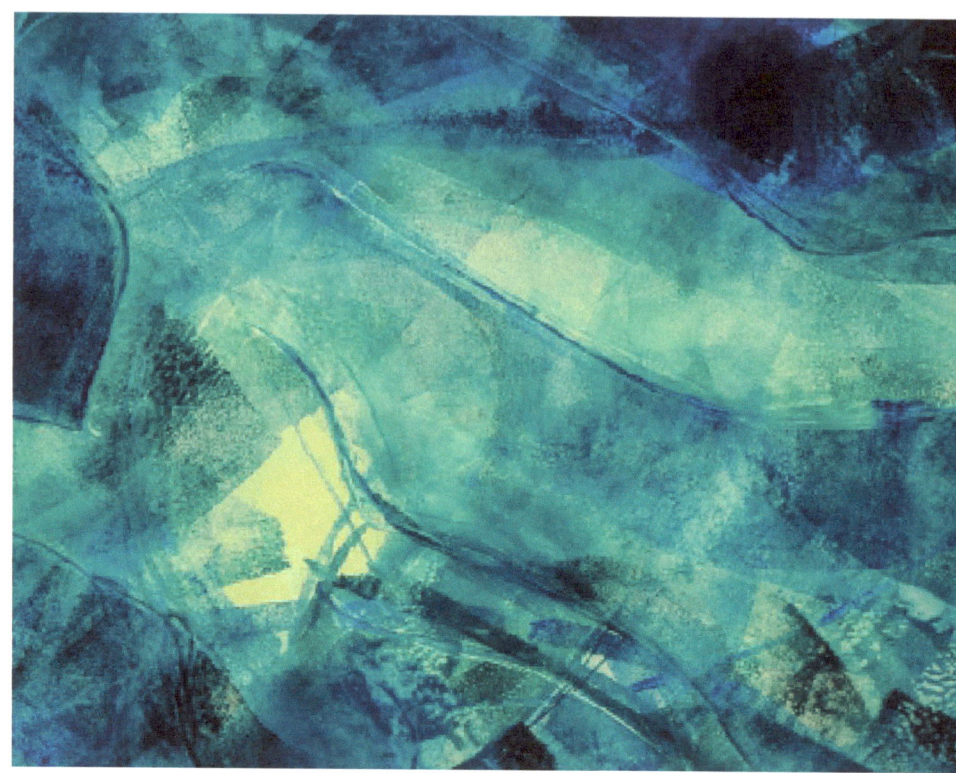

Breathe, repeat an affirmation and move.
Give life to your vision
as you re-create yourself
through the power of neuroplasticity.

SUSAN

Mudra is a Sanskrit word meaning 'closure' or 'seal.' Mudras are symbolic hand gestures used in yoga, and have an effect on the energy flow of the body. The term originated in Hindu culture. The mudras we have selected to represent each chakra have grown out of our thoughtful experimentation.

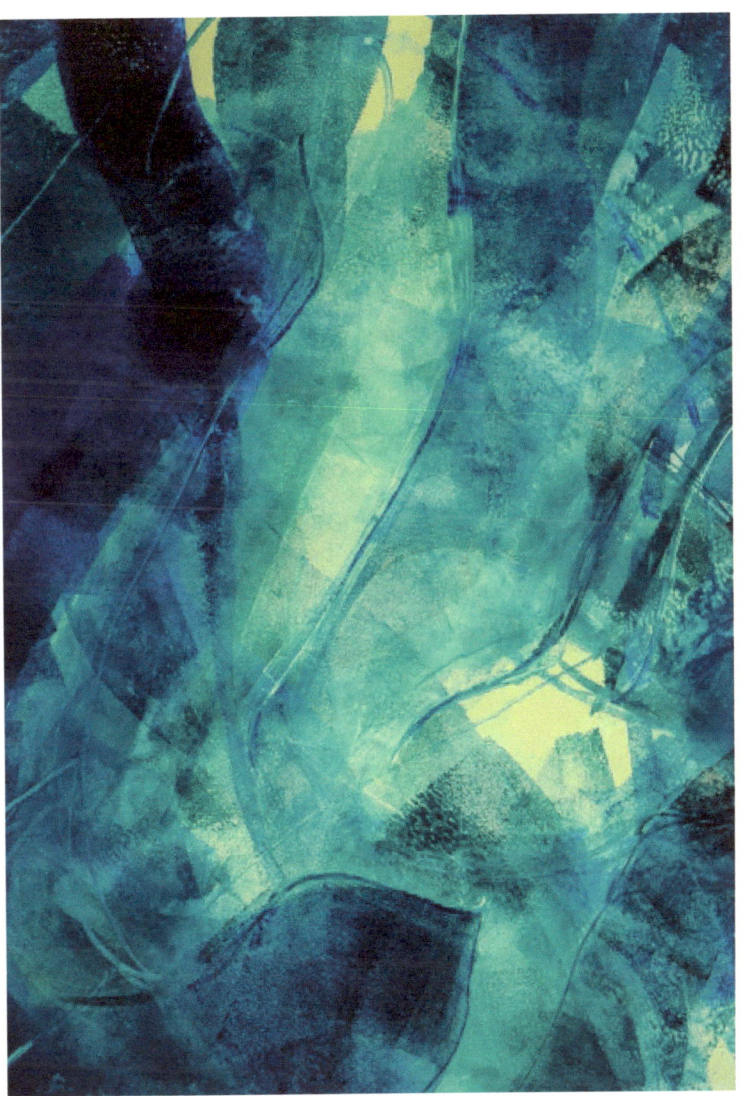

How the chakras are organized in this book

We have organized this book to be used by nyone, experienced or not in yoga. Our intention is to enable you to better understand the relevance of the chakras, and how practicing our simple meditation can invigorate and balance your life.

The description of each chakra includes:

- The Sanskrit name, its meaning and color
- Artistic representations for each chakra
- Location in the body
- Associated organs and glands
- Impact
- Affirmations and mantra
- A selected quote
- A demonstration of each chakra gesture

This format enables the reader to access the series of mudras that represent each chakra, and practice them with specific affirmations. The series can be done once or repeatedly, with the breath, and/or with an affirmation, said silently or out loud.

Gratitude concludes the series.

1. Root Chakra
Muladhara

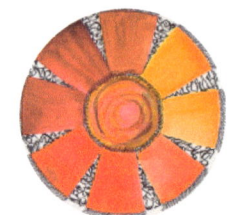

Color - Red

The word *Muladhara* breaks down into two Sanskrit words: Mula meaning 'root' and Adhara, which means 'support' or 'base.'

Located at the base of the spine, the pelvic floor, and the first three vertebrae.

Organs and Glands: anus, lower intestines, reproductive glands, kidneys.

Impact: grounds, roots and stabilizes weight and energy, nourishes legs and feet, stimulates the elimination of toxins.

Affirmation or Mantra:
I am becoming well grounded and balanced.

Mudra: hands on thighs, palms down; press palms gently into thighs to ground tailbone and pelvis (root into earth).

Quote:
"There is deep wisdom within our very flesh, if we can only come to our senses and feel it." Elizabeth A. Behnke

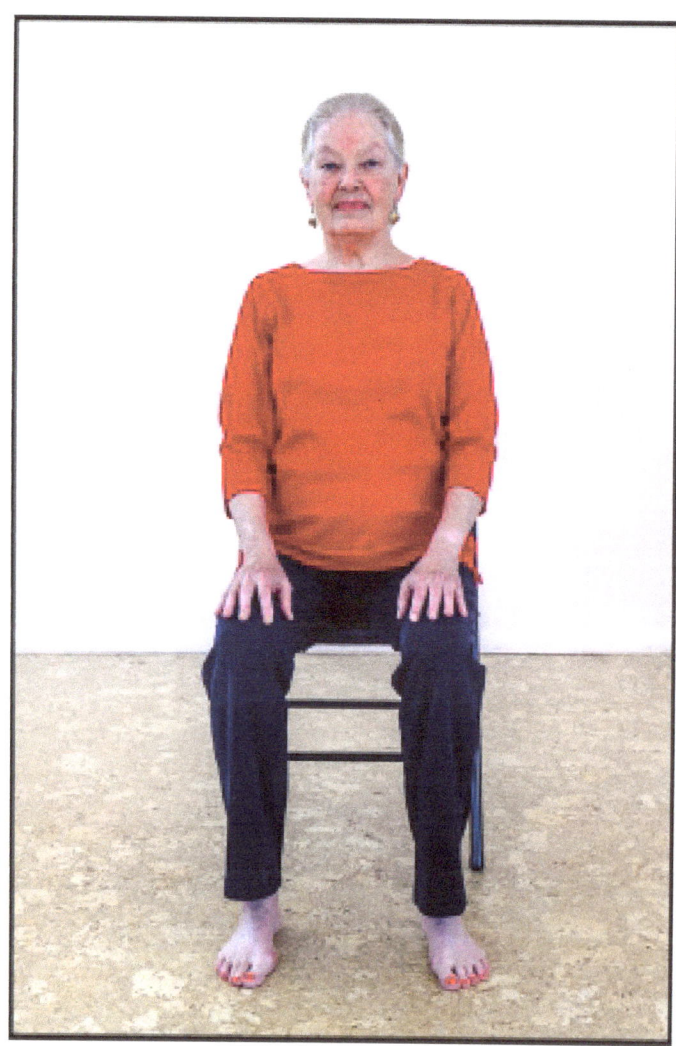

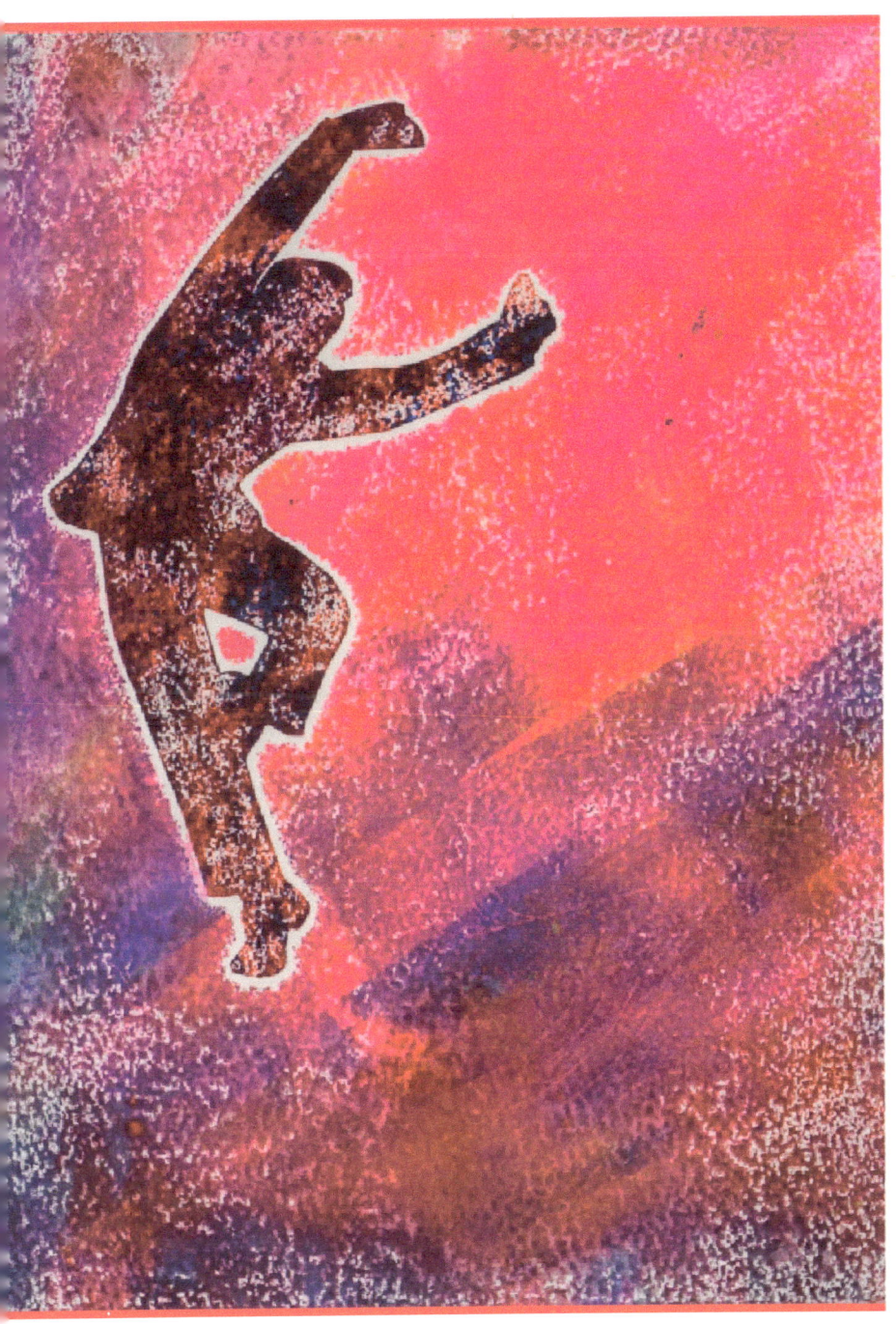

Some things you might like to know about the root chakra

The root chakra is responsible for our sense of safety and security. Balancing the root chakra creates the solid foundation for opening the other six chakras. It sets our foundation for all actions, including the positions of lying, sitting and standing.

The root chakra is comprised of whatever grounds you, and provides stability in your life. This includes your basic needs such as food, water, shelter, and emotional and physical safety.

If there is an imbalance in the root chakra you may experience anxiety, fears or nightmares. Physical imbalances may manifest as problems in the colon, with elimination, or with lower back, leg or foot issues. In men, prostate problems may occur. Eating disorders may also be a sign of a root chakra imbalance.

Establish your foundation to grow and expand your life

2. Sacral Chakra
Svadhisthana

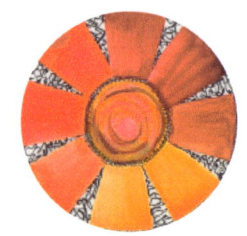

Color - Orange

The word *svadhisthana* can be translated as 'the dwelling place of the self'

Located in the lower abdomen, around the sacral bone behind and above the pubic bone in front, below the navel; it encompasses the genital region and the hypogastric plexus.

Organs and Glands: adrenal glands, sexual organs, bladder, kidneys, gall bladder, spleen, small intestines; regulates immune system.

Impact: sexual energy center, individual creativity, fertility, reproduction, bladder function.

Affirmation or Mantra:
I am a thinking, creative being and manifest vitality and sexual health.

Mudra: hands on thighs, palms face upward; press backs of hands gently into thighs.

Quote:
"Emotion always has its roots in the unconscious and manifests itself in the body." Irene Claremont de Castillejo

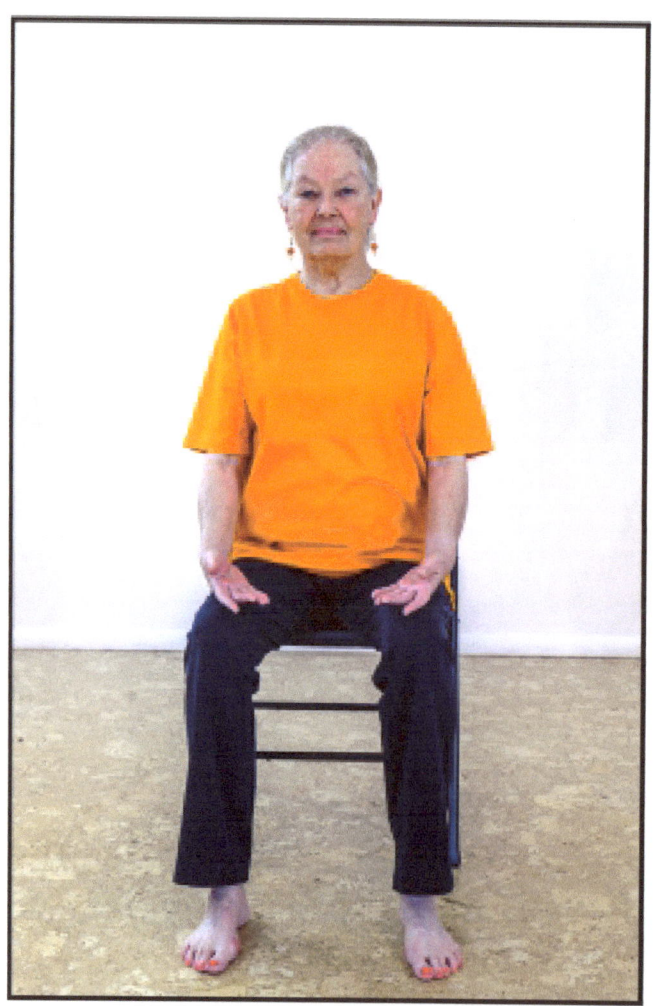

Some things you might like to know about the sacral chakra

The second chakra is known as the creativity and sexual chakra. When it is in balance, feelings of wellness, abundance, pleasure and joy will be experienced. When this chakra is out of balance, emotional instability, fear of change, sexual dysfunction, depression or addictions may be experienced.

The potential to create is within each of us. We don't need to be artists to create.

Creativity starts with curiosity, deep engagement, problem solving, dreaming and imagining; it also involves improvisation. It takes one into a timeless space where ideas, actions and possibilities are explored and new discoveries are made. From here we can see things from many different perspectives, rather than just one.

"Imagination is more important than knowledge."
Albert Einstein

Be playful and retain your ability to see things as new

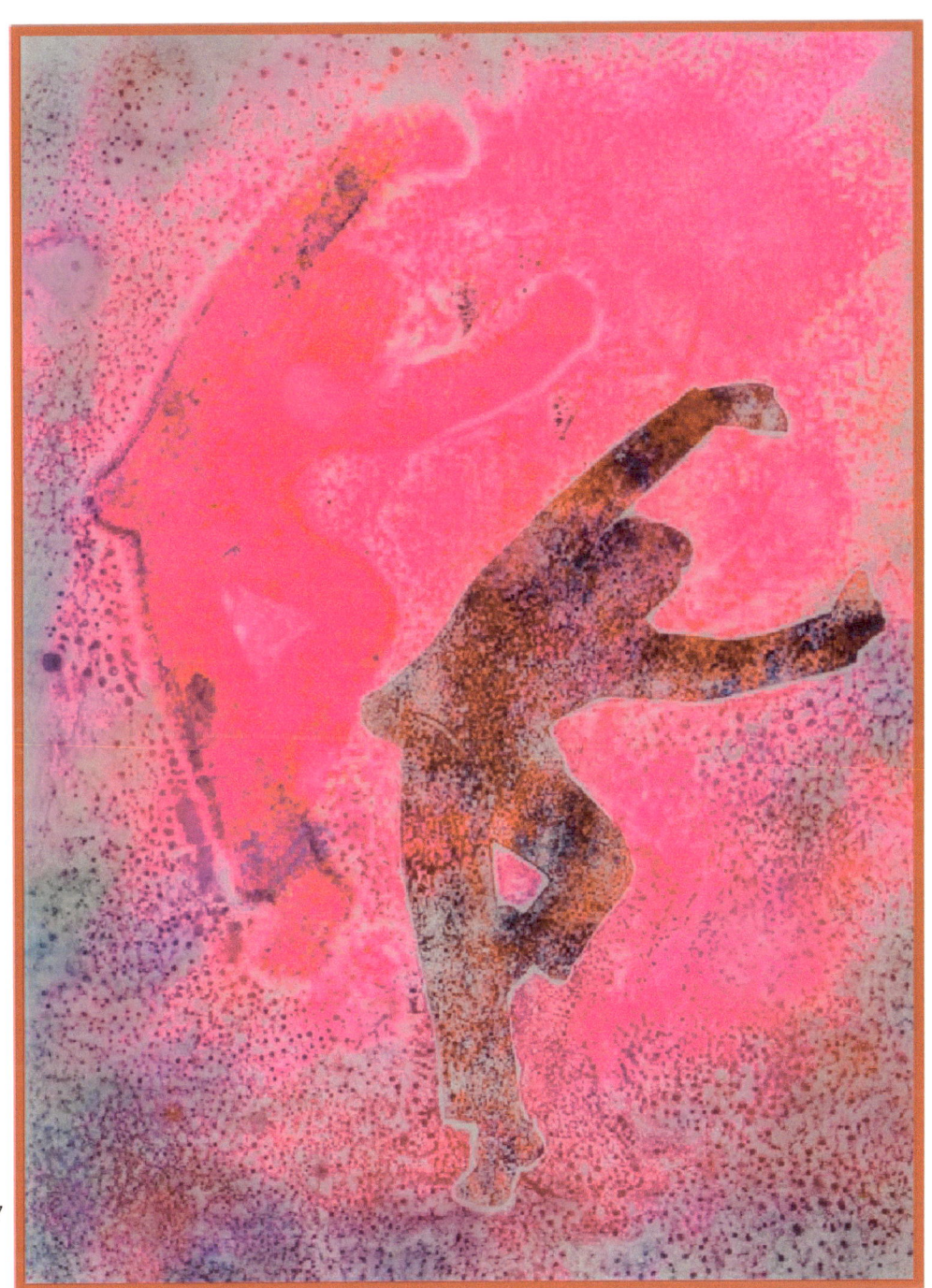

3. Solar Plexus Chakra
Manipura

Color - Yellow

The term *manipura* means 'lustrous gem.'

Located around the navel in the area of the solar plexus, it extends upward to the breastbone area.

Organs and Glands: stomach, liver, small intestines, esophagus, pancreas; regulates metabolism and digestion.

Impact: where our ego resides, sense of self esteem and confidence, commitment, emotional boundaries, supports drive to manifest ideas.

Affirmation or Mantra:
I am becoming calm, confident and capable.

Mudra: make a firm, but gentle fist with the left hand and place it over the belly; cover the closed fist with the right hand, bow the head slightly.

Quote:
"Every time you don't follow your inner guidance, you feel a loss of energy, loss of power, a sense of spiritual deadness."
Shakti Gawain

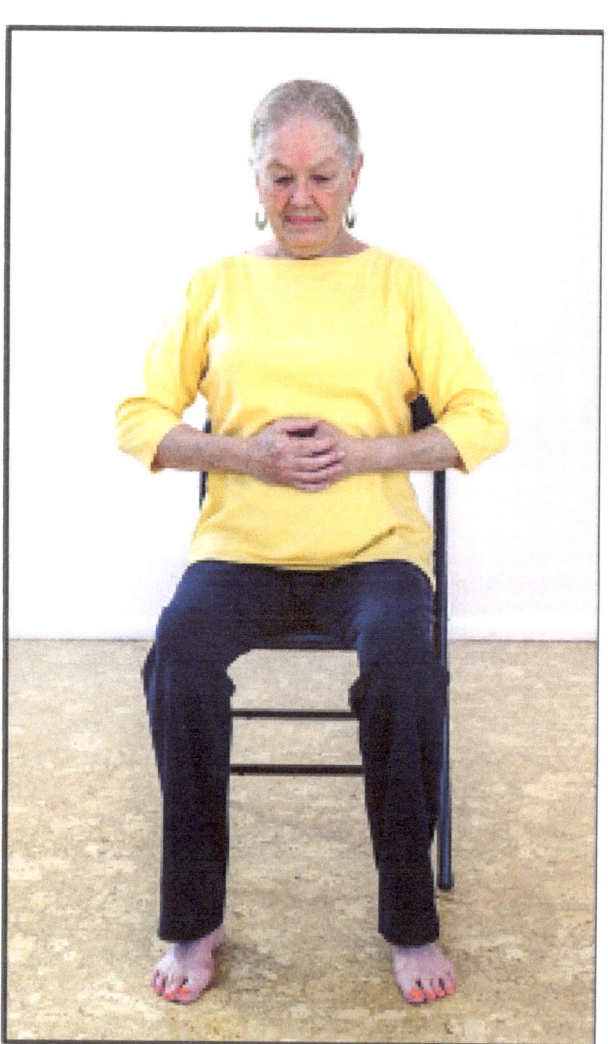

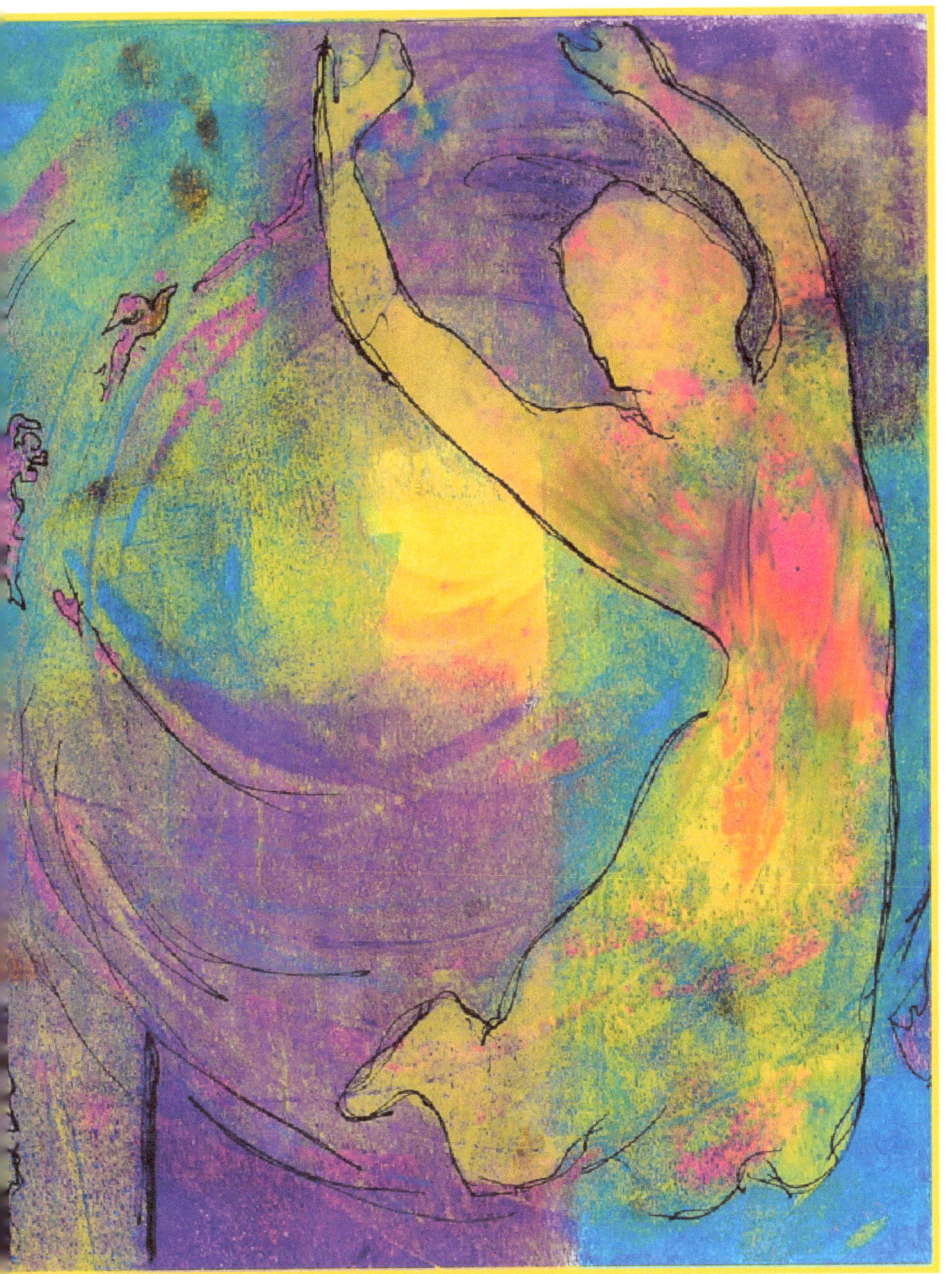

Some things you might like to know about the solar plexus chakra

A source of personal power, the solar plexus chakra impacts our self-esteem, core physical strength, our emotions and our abilty to transform.

When you feel self-confident, have a strong sense of purpose, and are selfmotivated, your third chakra is open and healthy. If this chakra is out of balance, you can suffer from low self-esteem, have difficulty making decisions, and may have anger or control issues.

Notice how you feel when you experience a loss, a change, or make a choice . This chakra will feel balanced when you make appropriate decisions regarding a situation - a queasiness or feeling of nausea may indicate that the decision is wrong

Trust your gut instinct!

4. Heart Chakra
Anahata

Color - Green

The Sanskrit word for the fourth chakra is *anahata*, meaning 'unstruck' or 'unhurt.' This suggests that one can get stuck beneath the hurts and grievances of past experiences.

However, through awareness you can contact a pure and spiritual place where no hurt exists.

Located at the center of the chest, it also governs the lymphatic system.

Organs and Glands: heart, lungs, esophagus, thymus, breasts; regulates metabolism.

Impact: strong emotions related to love, heartbreak, grief, pain, freedom, kindness, compassion; impacts lungs and breathing.

Affirmation or Mantra:
I am becoming kind and compassionate. I forgive myself and others.

Mudra: raise both arms above head, palms facing and elbows straight.

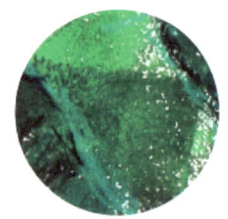

Quote:
"If you haven't any charity in your heart, you have the worst kind of heart trouble."

Bob Hope

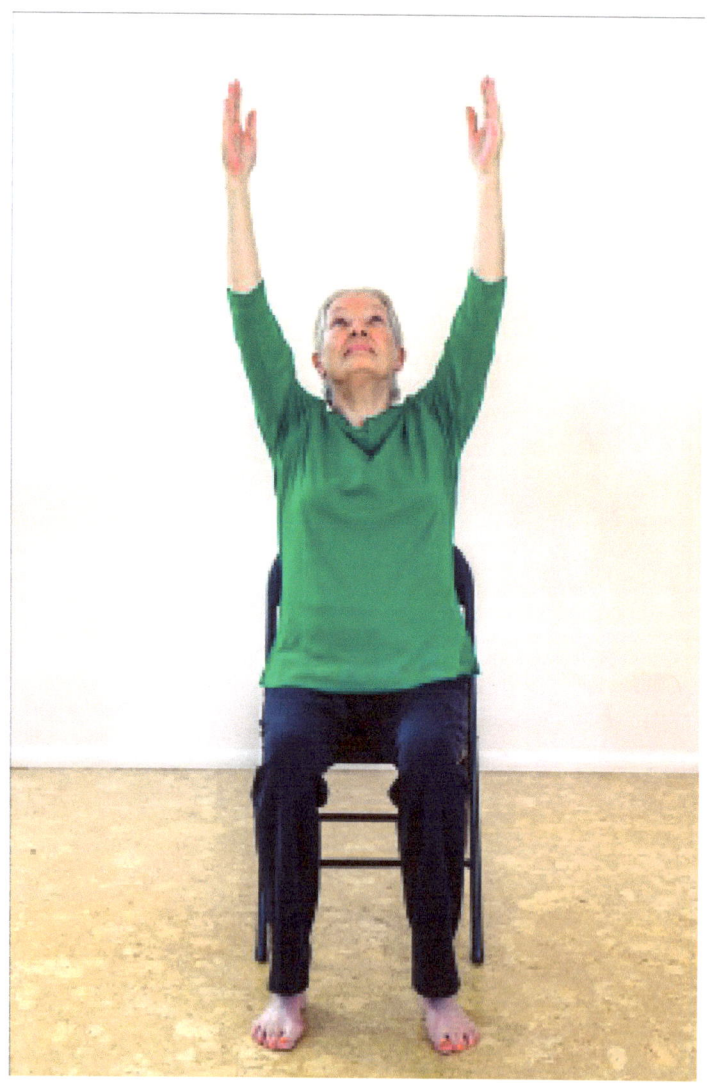

Some things you might like to know about the heart chakra

The fourth chakra represents the confluence of physical and spiritual energies. When your heart chakra is open, you are flowing with love and compassion, you are quick to forgive, and you accept others and yourself more easily. A closed heart chakra may lead to grief, anger, jealousy, fear of betrayal, and hatred toward yourself and others.

People can become stuck in a quagmire composed of grievances, sadness, resentment and blame. Such unresolved emotions are like quicksand – the more you struggle, the deeper you sink. They may have been hurt in the past by family members or acquaintances.
They may blame others, want revenge and stay angry in order to feel strong and remain victims. Unfortunately, these emotions are generated by fear, ignorance or hatred; all attest to a closed heart chakra.

When you are immersed in hurt feelings, whether past or present, you can choose to feel them fully, then let them go; or, hold onto them. By acknowledging them and releasing them, you will be able to open your heart again to people and experiences. Holding on to hurt harbors negative feelings and cuts you off from opportunities to love and serve. Letting go is about making a choice. Your mind and your ego may tell you otherwise, but it's as simple as choosing to forgive.

Letting go allows you to detach from the past and frees you to...

Live Your Now!

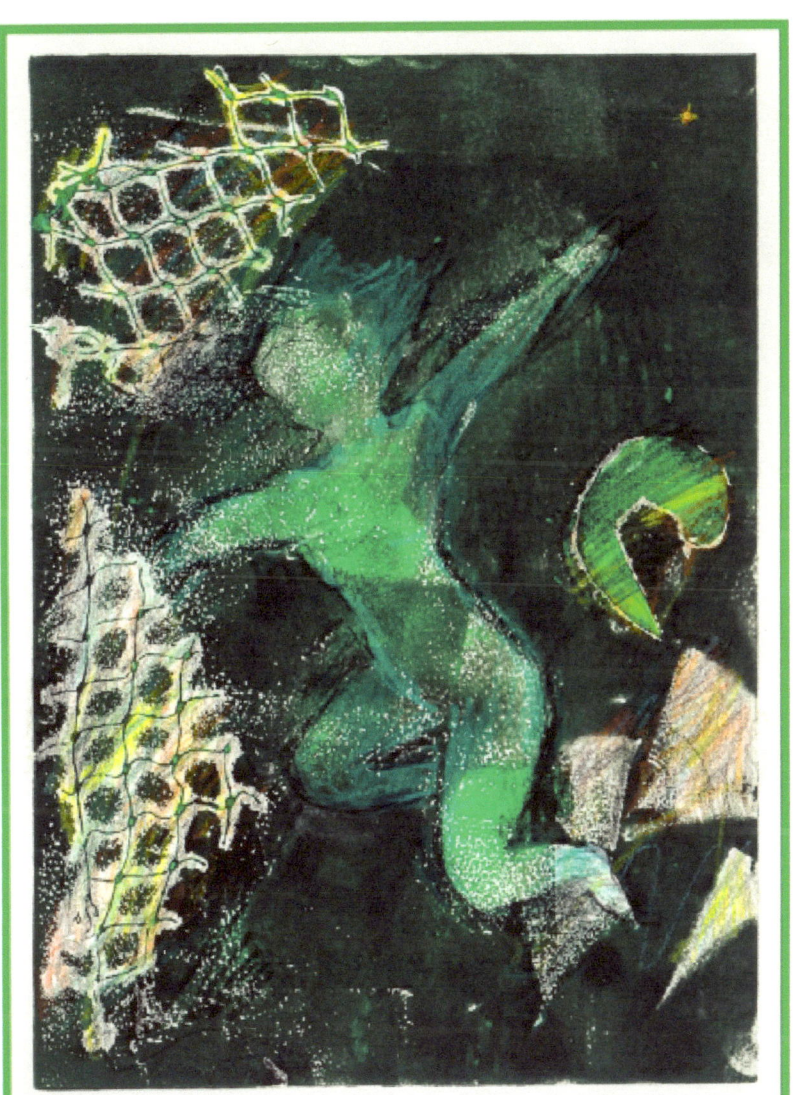

5. Throat Chakra
Vishuddha

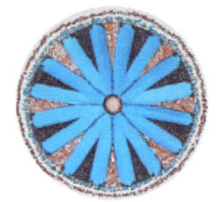

Quote:

"If you tell the truth you don't have to remember anything."

Mark Twain

Color – Blue – usually sky blue

Vishuddha is the first of the three spiritual chakras and means 'especially pure.'

Location: area around the throat, voice, thyroid, parathyroid, jaw, neck, mouth, tongue and larynx.

Organs and Glands: thyroid, bronchial tubes, vocal cords, respiratory system, mouth; connects to the lungs and esophagus, regulates body temperature and metabolism.

Impact: self-expression based on truth (satya) and compassion combined with wisdom, trustfulness, tension or lack of energy in vocal cords.

Affirmation or Mantra:
I strive to speak truthfully, guided by wisdom and compassion.

Mudra: open both arms out to side in a high diagonal, palms facing upward.

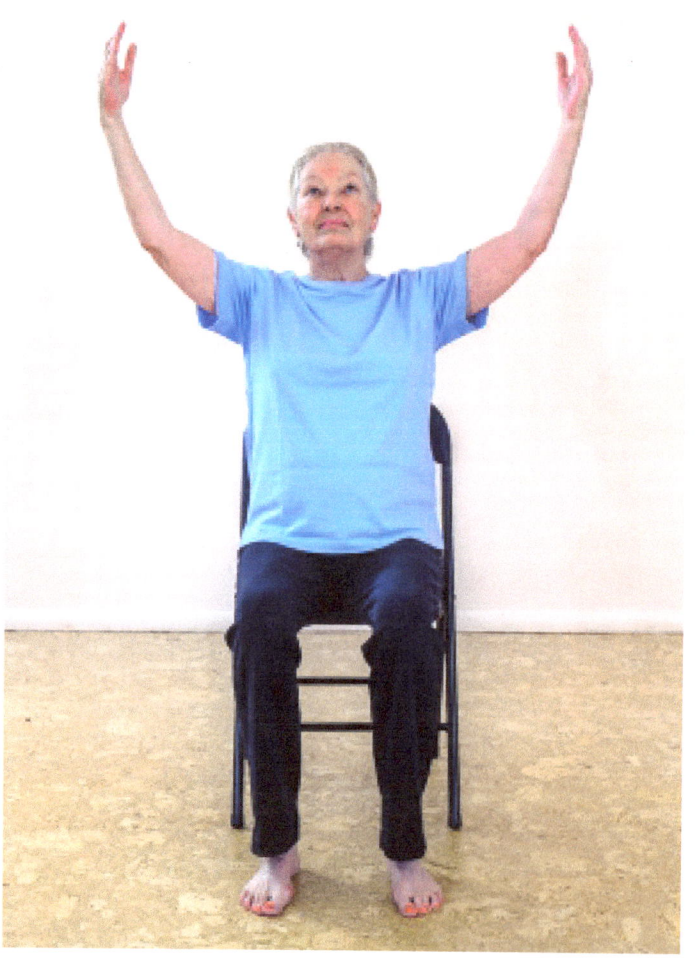

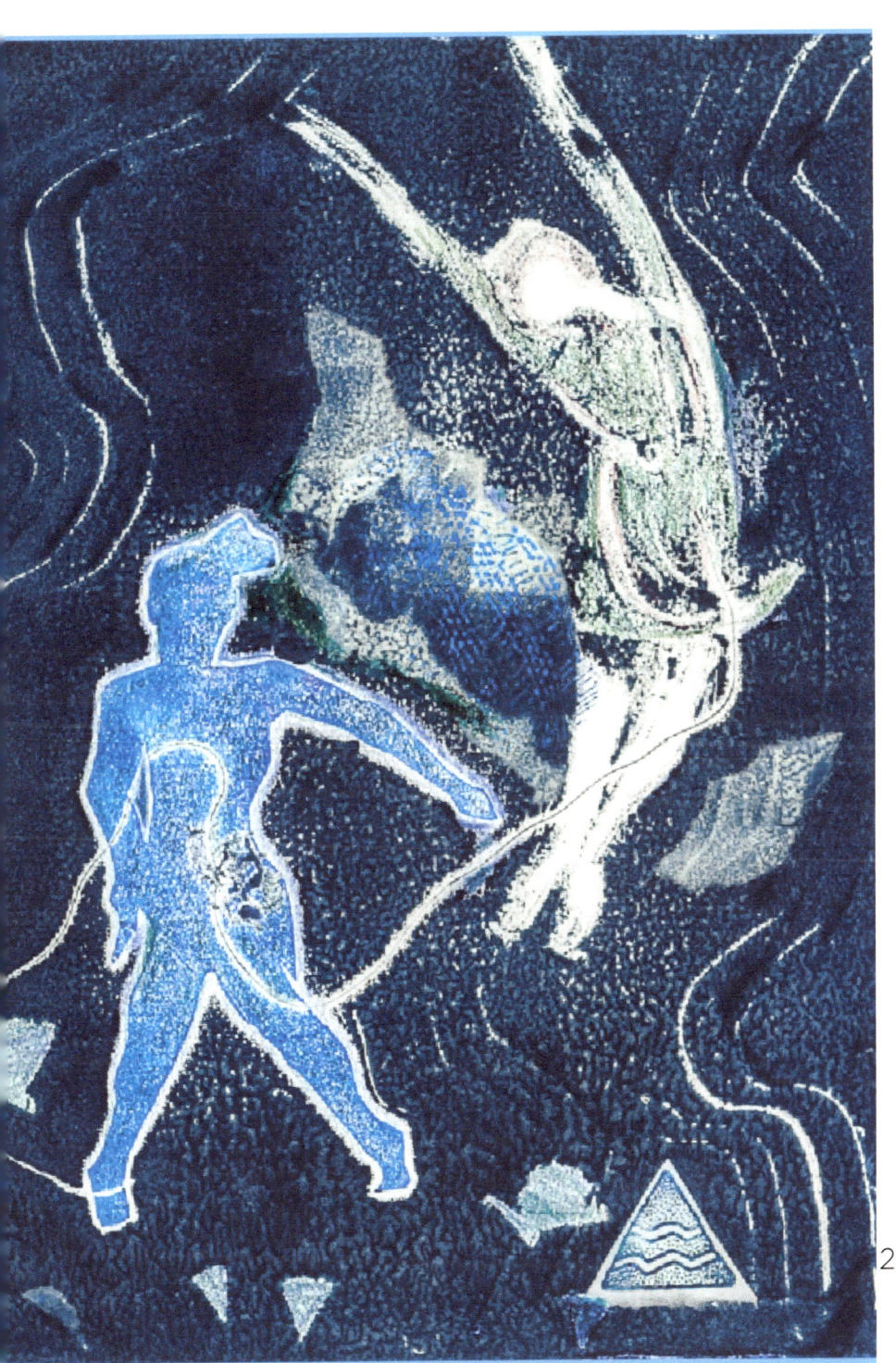

Some things you might like to know about the throat chakra

To be open and aligned in the fifth chakra is to speak, listen, and express yourself at an elevated form of communication. The highest form of this is to speak from a place of truth rather than speaking from a place of fear; or trying to say what you think is wanted or acceptable. It is better to express yourself truthfully rather than setting yourself up for a series of untruths. Think about whether you need to say something, how you can say it honestly, and whether you can be kind and compassionate with your words. It is also important to avoid being opinionated and judgmental.

Another big aspect of speaking and expressing yourself is to allow others to do the same; be a good listener and witness rather than be a commentator, critic or evaluator.

Speak your truth with kindness and wisdom

6. Third Eye Chakra
Ajna

Color – Indigo Blue or Violet

Ajna means 'beyond wisdom,' and leads to an inner knowledge that will guide you if you let it.

Location: on the forehead between the two brows.

Organs and Glands: brain, eyes, ears, pituitary and pineal glands, head, and lower part of the brain.

Impact: connects to the frontal cortex of the brain, impacts intuition, imagination and wisdom, helps focus on seeing The Big Picture, helps us to access information from various sources, connects our inner world with the outer world of reality, extrasensory perception.

Affirmation or Mantra:
I am open to using all my perceptions to make wise decisions.

Mudra: arms lower slightly and elbows bend into the waist; touch the forefinger and thumb of each hand (jnana mudra – means knowledge)

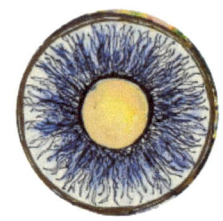

Quote:

"It's not what you look at that matters, it's what you see."

Henry David Thoreau

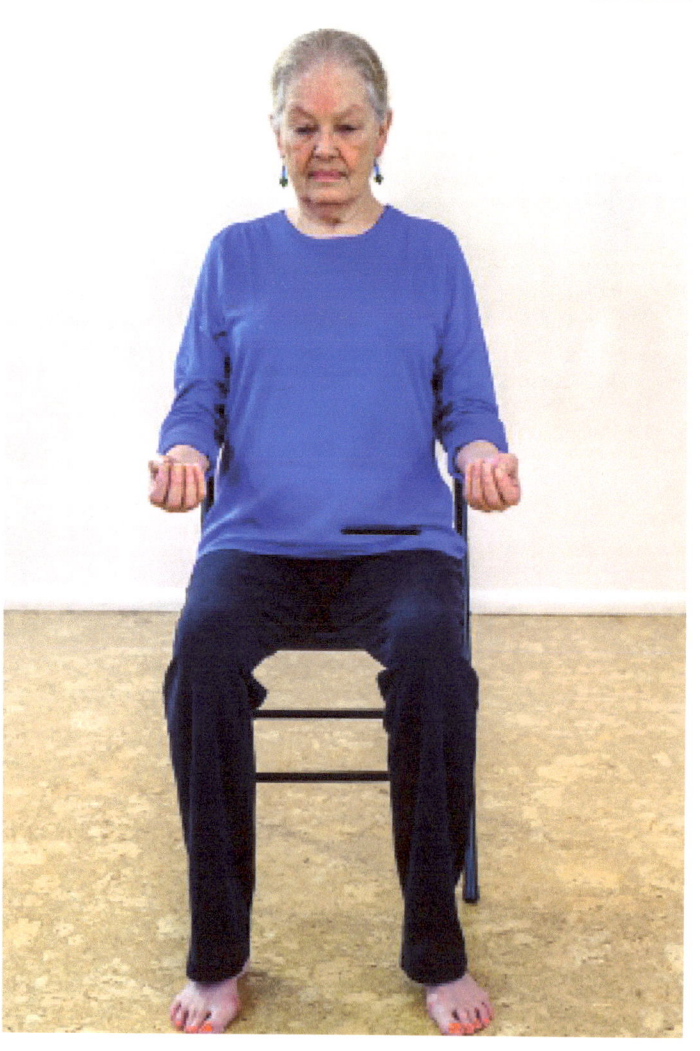

Some things you might like to know about the third eye chakra

The world is experienced through the five senses – sight, touch, smell, taste and hearing. The third eye chakra is a combination of all the information provided by the senses, kinesthetic information and the mind. It is the center of intuition and wisdom. An open sixth chakra enables clairvoyance, telepathy, lucid dreaming, expanded imagination and visualization . By tapping into intuition, it allows us to trust our perceptions, bypassing misleading clues and false information. Listening to our intuition hightens our sensitivity and guides us in making good decisions.

Trust your intuition

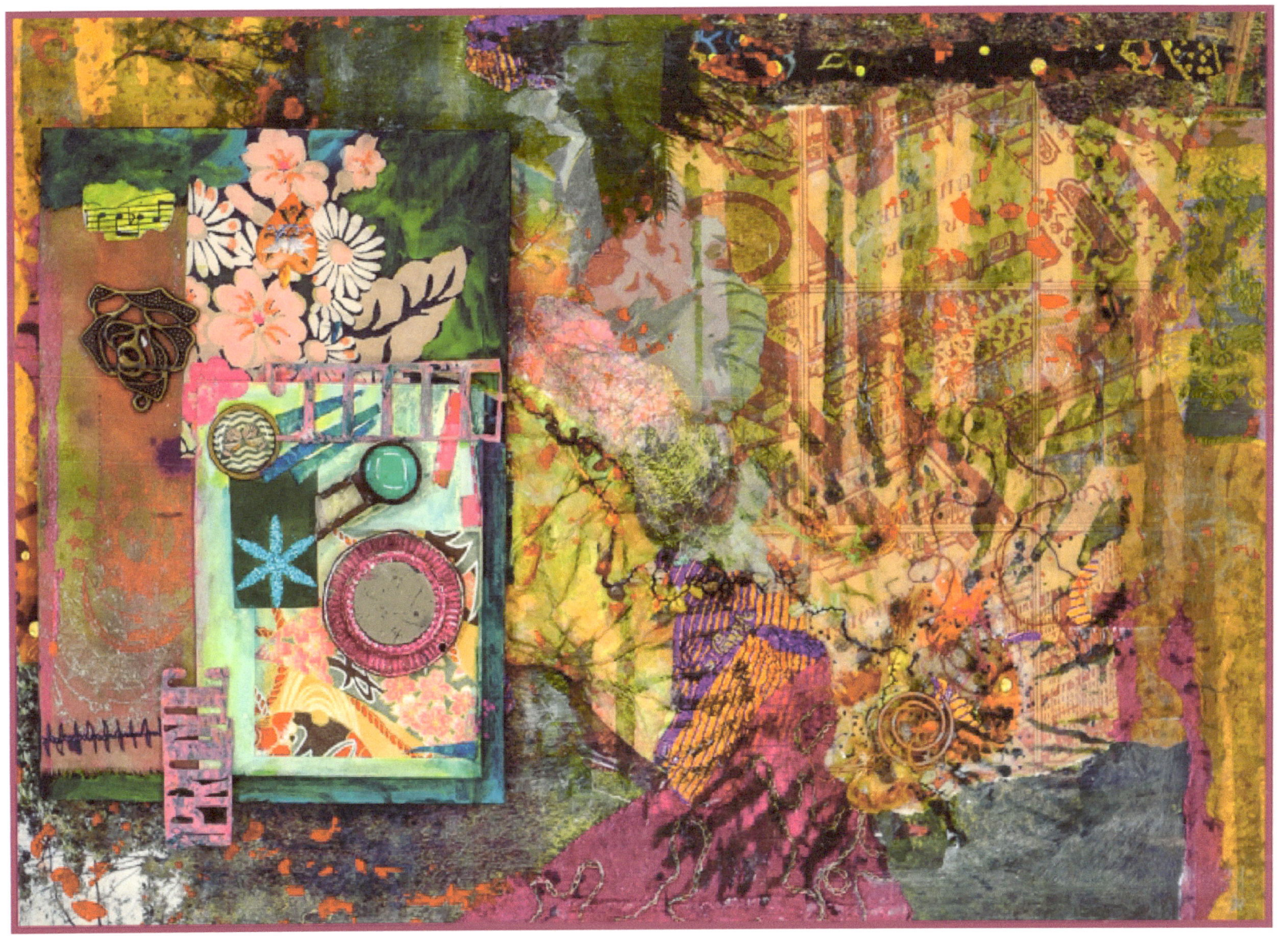

7. Crown Chakra
Sahasrara

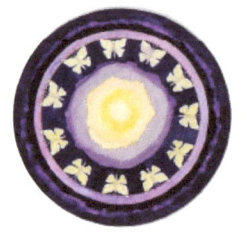

Color – White, light violet or delicate pink.

Sahasrara means 'lotus petals.' This chakra is often depicted as a lotus flower with open petals representing spiritual awakening . It is the center for trust, devotion, inspiration, contentment and optimism.

Located at the top, or even several inches above, the head or skull; can serve as an entry way for the Universa l Life Force to enter our awareness.

Organs and Glands: spinal cord, pineal gland, brain; regulates biological cycles including sleep.

Impact: connects us to our spirituality and bliss, giving access to the fields of energy that surround us.

Affirmation or Mantra:
I connect to universal energy to empower my life.

Mudra: lower both arms diagonally; press palms downward and extend the head upward.

Quote:
"We can be knowledgable with other men's knowledge, but we cannot be wiff with other men's wisdom."
   Michel de Montaigne

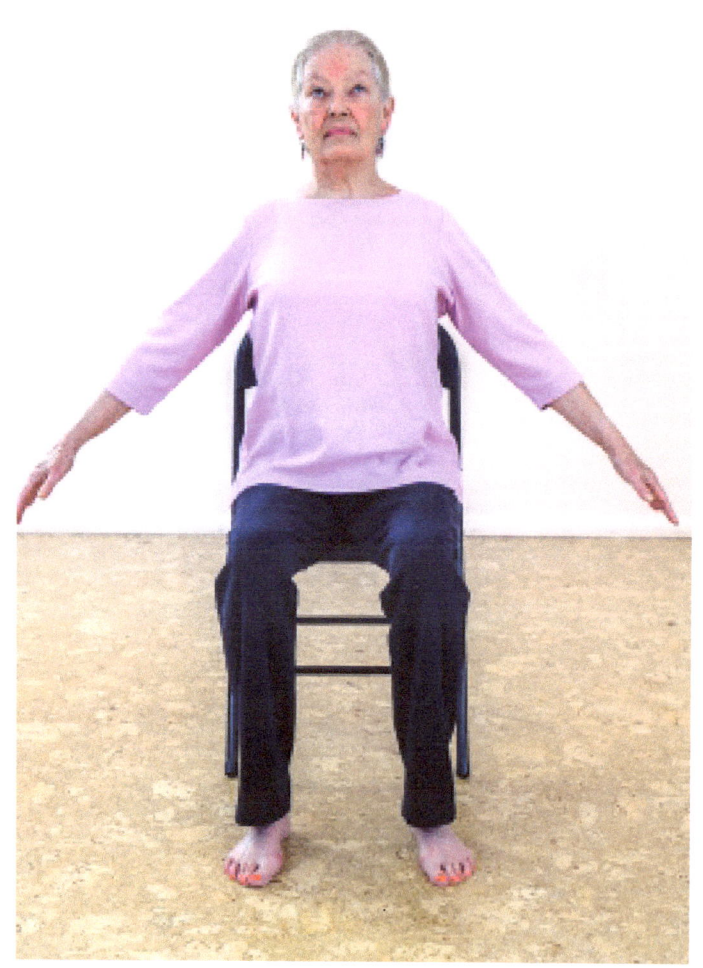

Some things you might like to know about the crown chakra

Think of the crown chakra as representing universal energy, similar to an ocean that ebbs and flows. As individuals, we are molecules of water – collectively we are an ocean. This is the chakra of deep connection to everything in life. Each of us is pure consciousness and each of us matters. We can rise into clouds and we can drop back to earth as rain.

It is also the center for a deeper connection within ourselves and with the 'Forces of Life' – that which is greater than ourselves. Each of us is pure consciousness, undivided and all expansive.

Silence and meditation are the most powerful and important ways to stimulate and open the seventh chakra.

**Expand your life -
connect to universal energy**

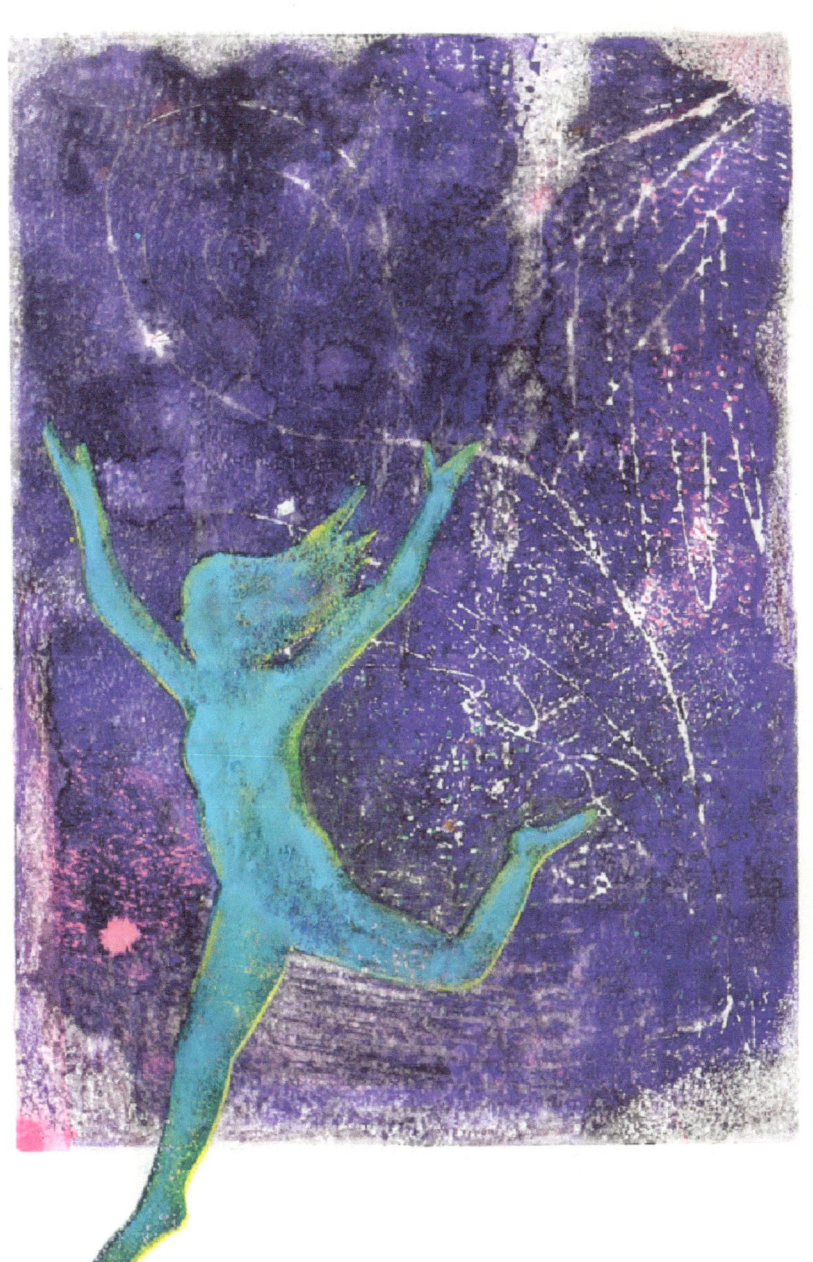

8. Gratitude
Dhanyosmi

Dhanyosmi is the art of expressing gratitude

Culminating Mudra: press palms together lightly at the heart center in a gesture of reverence (*anjali mudra* – to offer or celebrate). When we give gratitude, we honor ourselves, others, our experiences and life itself This position reminds us that all the chakras are connected and function in an integrated way for optimum mental, emotional, physical and spiritual health .

Affirmations or Mantras

I am open and available to all that is.
I am thankful for being alive.

I am thankful for the chance to create,
embrace and fulfill my life.

It is customary to end our meditations with these two words – *namaste* and *shanti*.

Namaste: *the divine light within me salutes the divine light within you.*

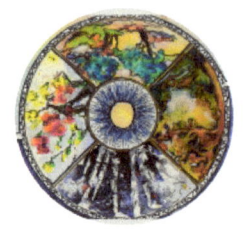

Shanti: *peace.*

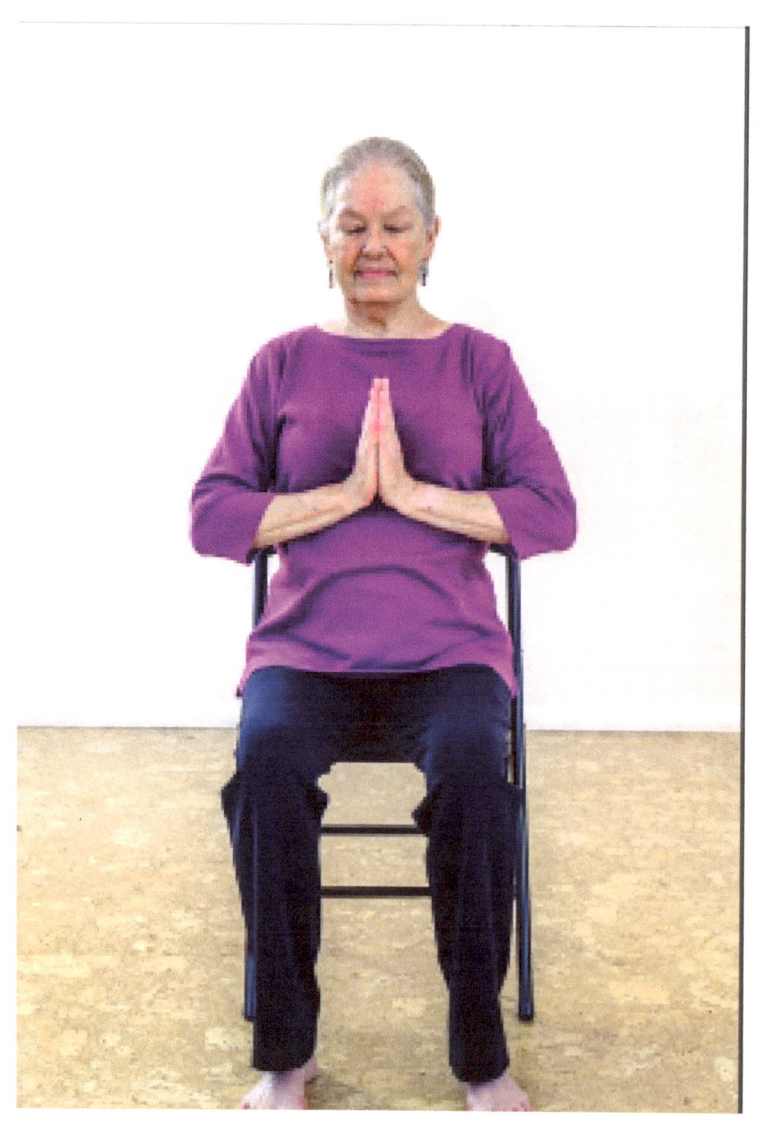

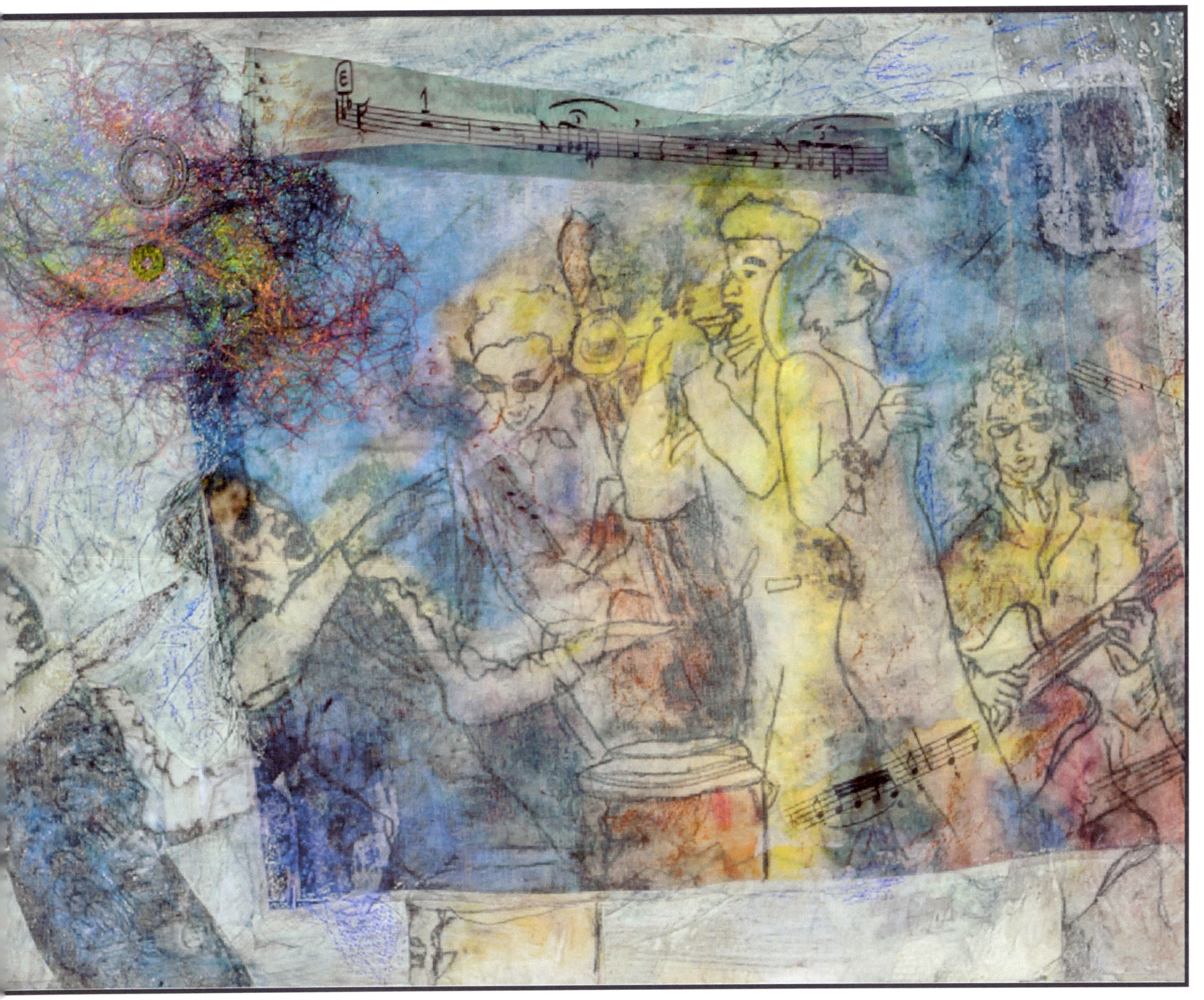

MUDRAS SITTING IN A CHAIR

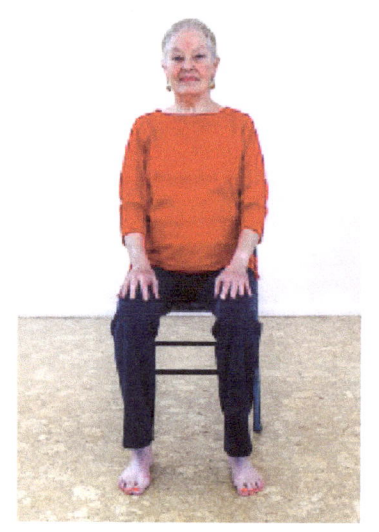
ROOT

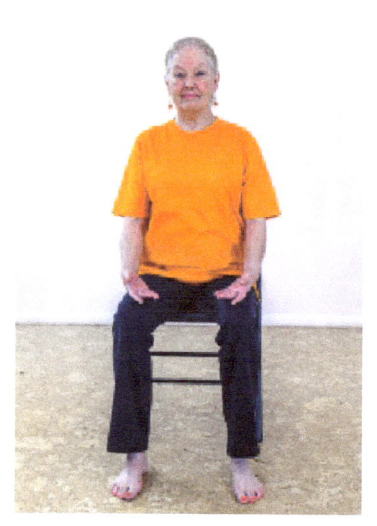
SACRAL

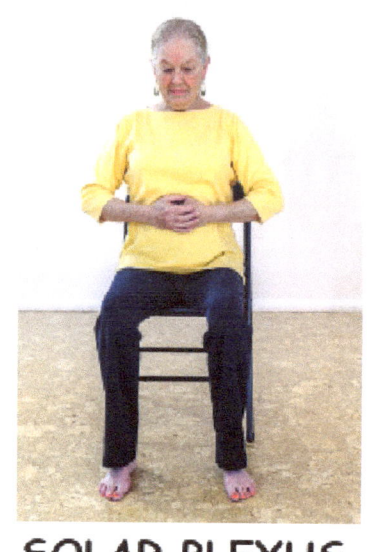
SOLAR PLEXUS

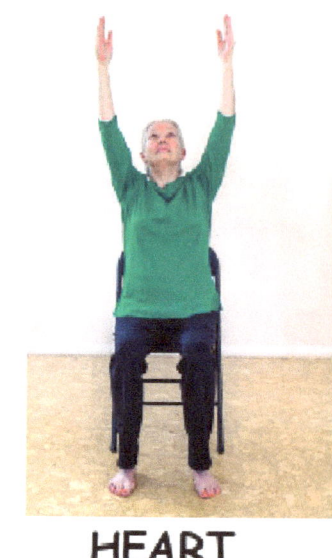
HEART

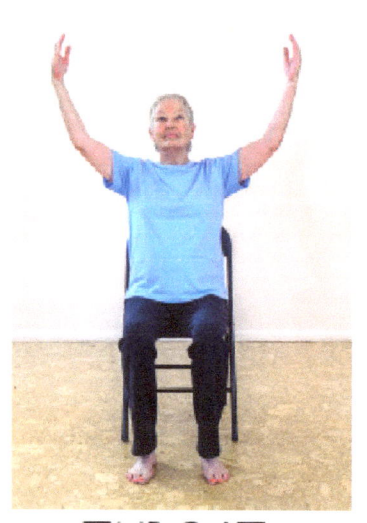
THROAT

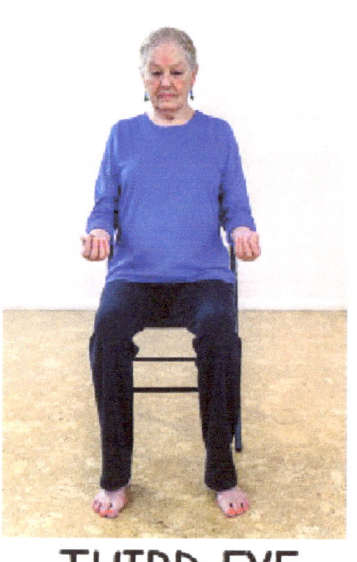
THIRD EYE

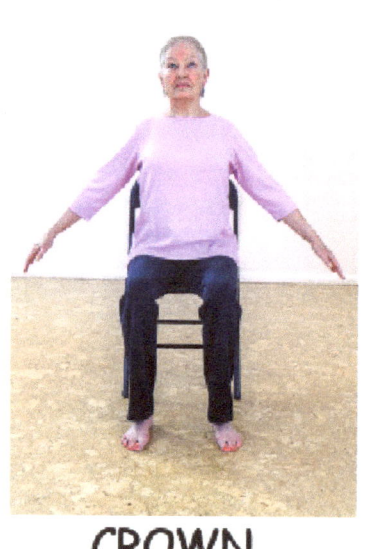
CROWN

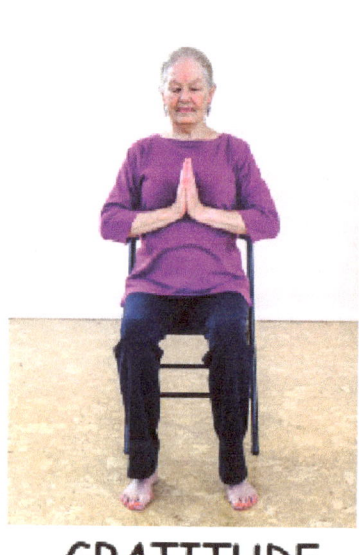
GRATITUDE

MUDRAS SITTING ON A BOLSTER

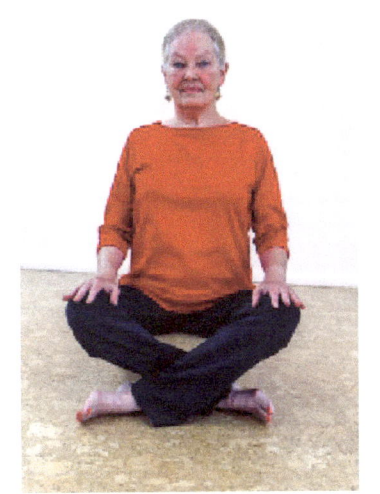
ROOT

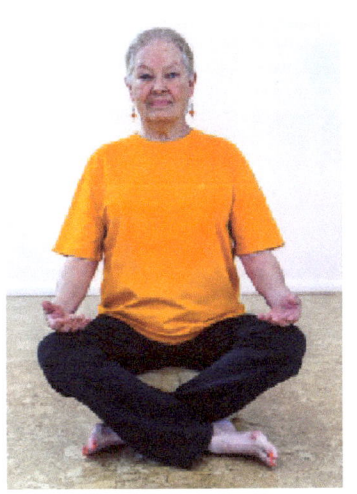
SACRAL

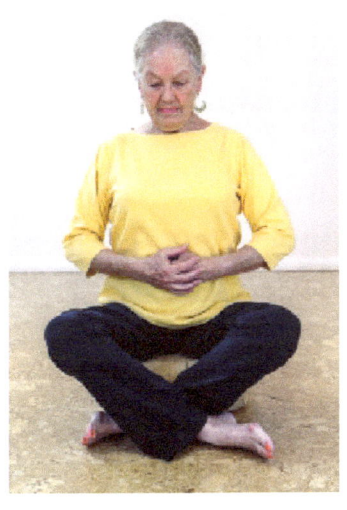
SOLAR PLEXUS

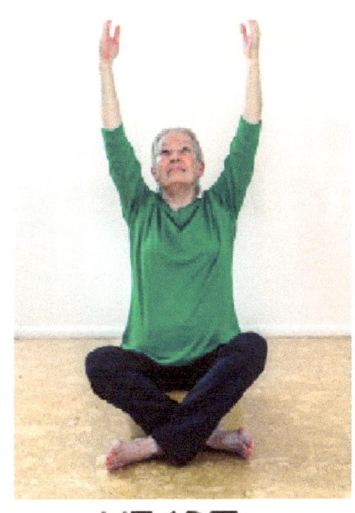
HEART

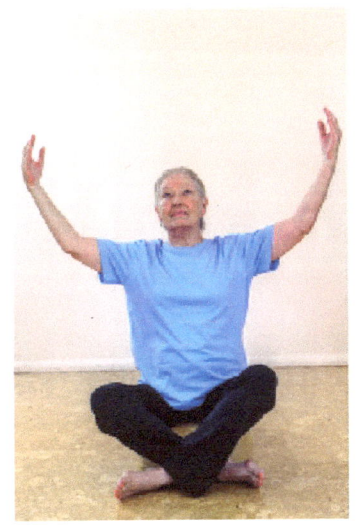
THROAT

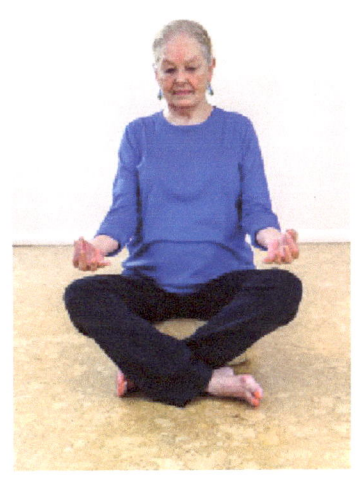
THIRD EYE

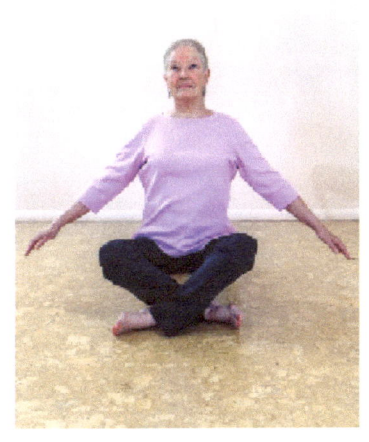
CROWN

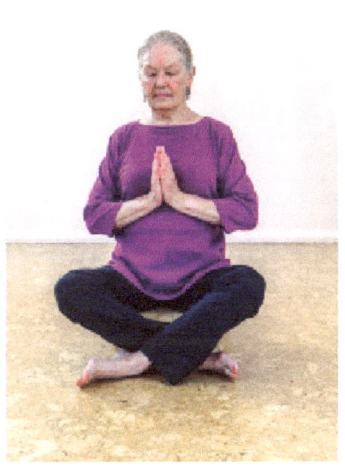
GRATITUDE

SUSAN'S PERSONAL STORY
How my Heart Chakra Opened

It is one thing to open up your heart when everything is going well and you are happy. It is quite another to open it when unexpected tragedy comes and shatters your world. This flings you into a nightmare that challenges your sanity and removes any degree of normalcy. When this happened to me, my very worst nightmare became a reality. I was given dramatic choice to make in a short moment - and the choice I made would change the course of my life. It determined whether I would become one of the walking dead or find a small glimmer of goodness, courage and hope within myself to hold onto.

My beautiful daughter, Julie, had just turned 19. Starting her first year in college, she had recently ended a long-time love relationship with her high school boyfriend, and was moving on in her life. She was an artistic, creative, strong and determined young woman. A few days after her birthday, her former boyfriend came to take her out for a long-promised ice cream to celebrate. Ten minutes after they drove off in her car along Sunset Boulevard - with him driving - they were both dead. My husband and I didn't learn about it for several hours until the police came to our door at 3:00 a.m. with the news. It felt like a nightmare had enveloped and held me hostage.

I couldn't escape. Just a side bar - while no drugs or alcohol were involved, there was still emotional volatility between them.

I don't wish to draw you any deeper into my grief, and there is no point going into the specifics. Julie's former boyfriend was someone I also loved. I knew him well since they were together for most of their teens, and he was often at our house. I felt double grief at their sudden deaths.

However, what I do wish to share is a dream I had. It wasn't so much a dream as a 'visitation.' About a week after their funerals he appeared before me. He was very emotional - devastated sobbing and asking for my forgiveness. As I saw and felt him there in my room, my heart opened and I felt deep love and compassion for him. I knew he would never do anything to purposefully hurt my daughter. I knew he was sincere in his remorse and in his request.

Without any hesitation, I forgave him - he immediately faded, disappearing into a void. I knew I had freed him from remaining earthbound. In forgiving him, I had allowed him to move on.

What I didn't know then was that my forgiveness freed me as well. My eyes popped open. I abruptly sat up in bed, fully awake, my heart beating rapidly. I woke my husband and told him what had happened. Although roused from a deep sleep, he listened without judgment and with love. I told him that I surprised myself when I forgave the young man without hesitation. I instantaneously experienced an enormous relief, followed by a feeling of peaceful calm (santosha). I knew that they had both survived their physical deaths. I had been given a gift of insight and understanding that was profound.

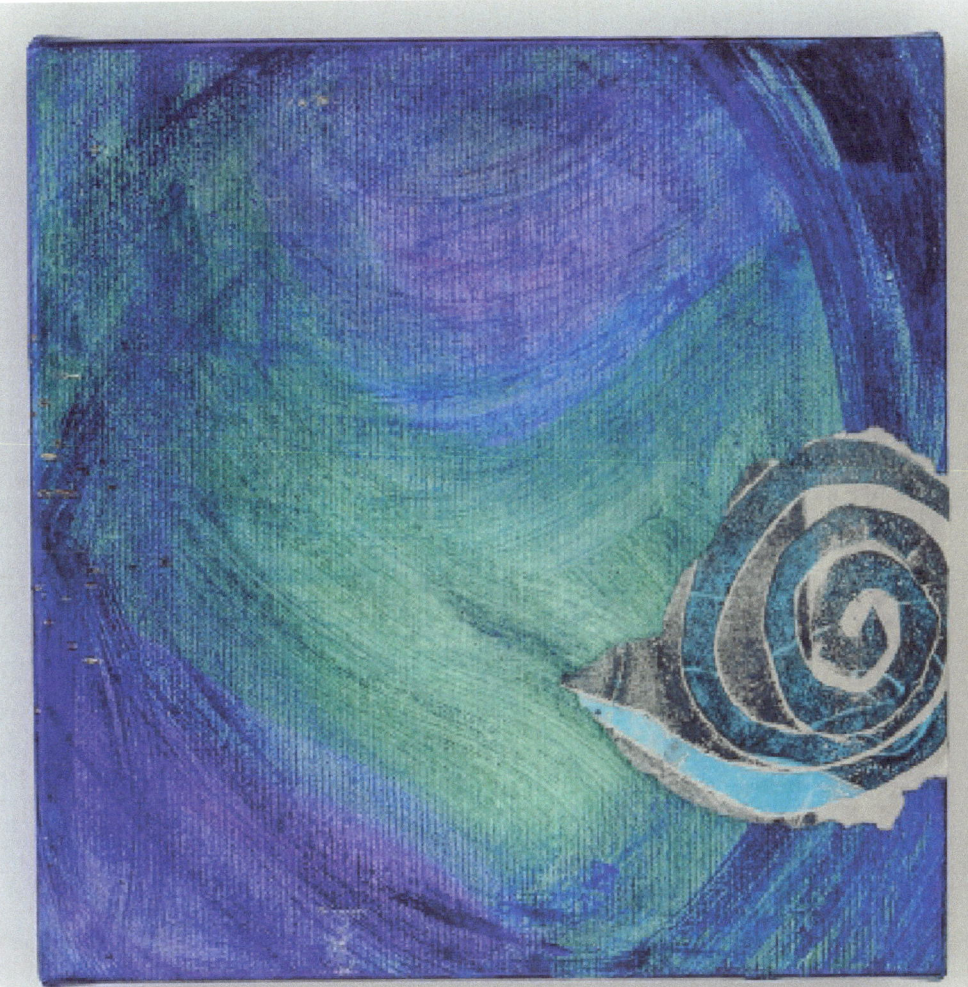

This encounter was a turning point for me - I shifted my view from what I had lost to all that I had been given. As my oldest daughter, Julie taught me to be a mother. We went through all of the key stages of the mother-daughter relationship. I had the privilege of knowing her, guiding her, learning from her - and nothing could take those gifts from me - not even death.

That dream opened up a portal for me to enter a world of heightened awareness and transformation. Of course, the healing process has continued formany years; I am still mining the gifts buried deep in my cells. But, this was the experience that gave me the insight and courage to not only recover from this loss, but to expand in order to live more fully.

Everyone experiences change, loss, and difficult challenges at different points in their life journey. Personal losses cannot be compared. Each person must find the resources within themselves to deal with change. There is a choice - blame others, grieve forever, remain trapped and bound by the chains of your own agreement to remain a victim; or, feel the pain, view the situation with courage, release the crippling emotions and set an intention to heal. This is the only way you can fully embrace the rest of your moments (no one knows how many moments you will be given) and give fully to the people who are still with you. It is about forgiveness and opening up your heart.

Live Your Now!

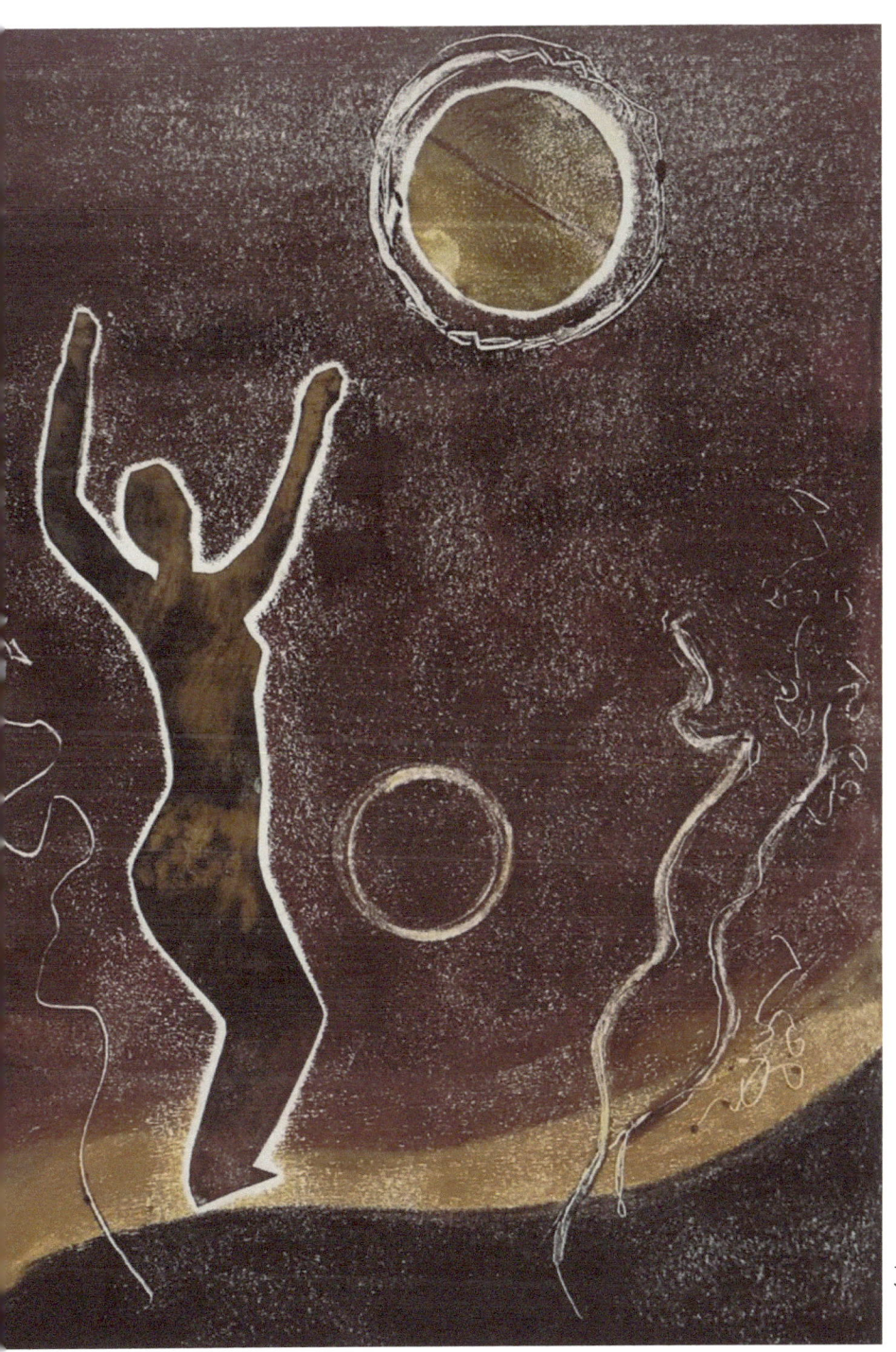

GLIMPSES INTO EMPOWERING YOUR LIFE

This new edition of *Live Your Now* features a series of 12 essays on different topics of life, using the lens of yoga. Susan wrote the first eleven, and her husband Paul wrote the final one. Each has drawn from the principles and teaching of yoga, referencing their more than eighty years each of living. Think of these 12 works as a dozen eggs. Each is filled with the potential to hatch something new – unique to you and your interests in moving towards a more joyful, peaceful, purposeful and responsible life.

Several will challenge you to expand your viewpoint. Some will entice you to re-examine your way of approaching things. And a few might inspire and motivate you towards positive change!

Enjoy!

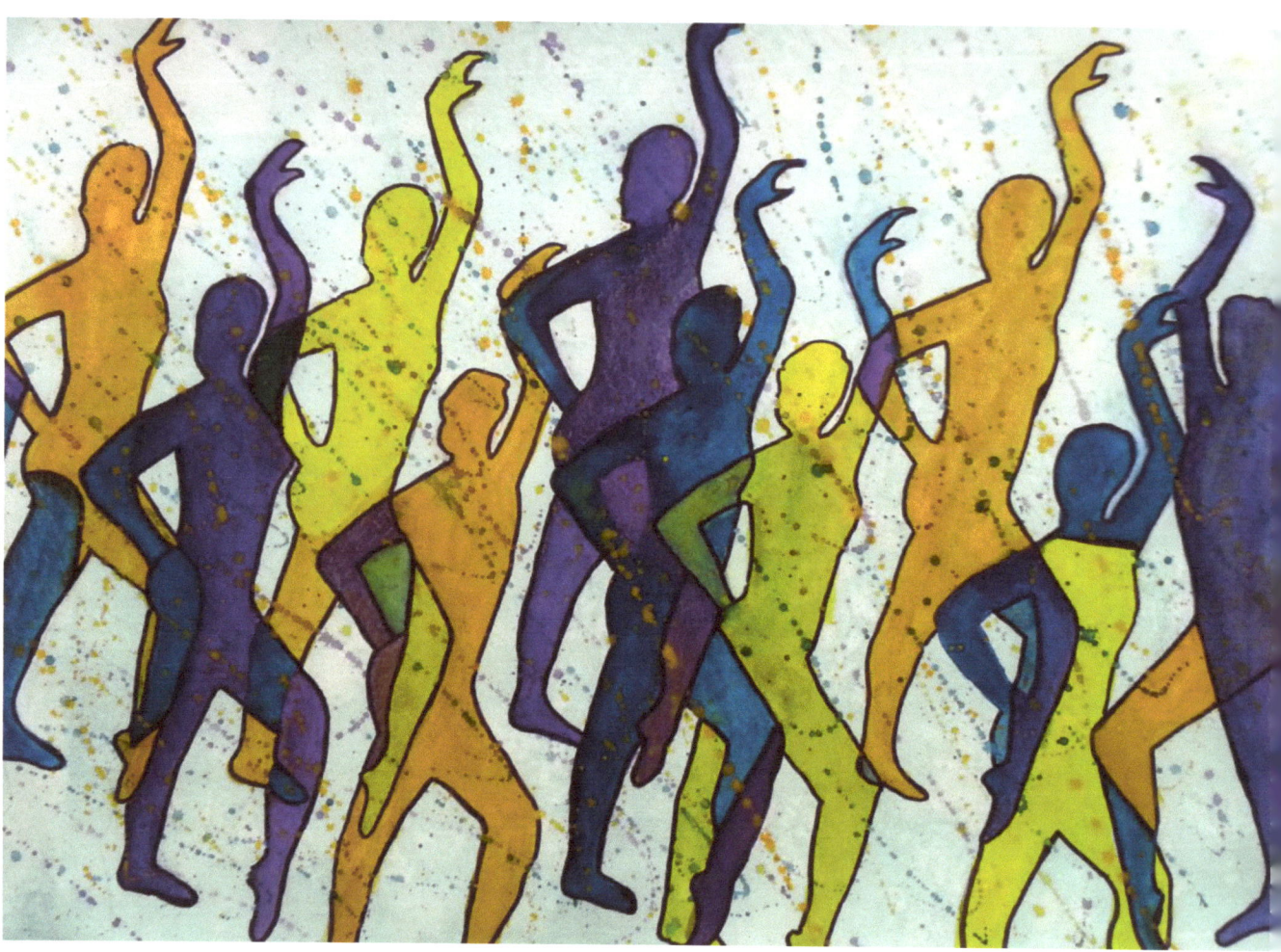

#1 Don't Ever Give Up!

How many of us put up our own **Stop Signs** in life?

"Stop! –You are too young!"
      "Stop! –You aren't good enough!"
           "Stop! –You aren't smart enough!"
                "Stop! –You don't have any talent!"
                      "Stop! –You are a woman!"
                            "Stop! –You aren't tall (thin
                                  or pretty) enough!"

And, one characteristic that catches up with all of us -
"Stop! You are too old!"

Think about all the "Stops" that delayed, prevented, and moved you away from fulfilling your true self

Well, I stopped myself at many points along the way. At times it was a struggle to feel worthy of being happy and fulfilled. But, there was always a tiny flame within me that just wouldn't be blown out. We all have that flame within us that continues to burn, even as an ember, until we take our last breath and exit our body.

While you are still alive, it is possible to fan that ember or tiny flame - that little light within each of us! Remember the joyous song many of us sang in our youth, *"This little light of mine; I'm gonna let it shine!"*? Those words continue to replay themselves inside my heart and head whenever I face a dead-end.

I would imagine myself in a dark hole that I had dug. It was so dank and lonely that I brought in imaginary twinkle lights to brighten up my space. Eventually, I added more and more until one day I decided to claw my way up the side of my chasm, now complex and multi-layered. It was a big and exhausting struggle - but, something within me would not give up. Finally, I was able to reach the sunlight of day and the moonlight of night and resume my journey with some awe, curiosity and balance.

When I was 50, I designed a personal 25-year plan. At 69, I had accomplished all of it, so wrote a revised 5-year plan to take me to my 75th birthday. I decided to retire from a long career as a teaching dance artist and director of curriculum and training for a major arts institution. That never happened! I continued to work full time, but also signed up to do the 500 hours of training to quality as a certified yoga instructor, tackling the required rigorous study and practice. Of course, I was the oldest one in the group!

Surrounded by people in their 20s, 30s, and 40s - there was one 55 year old who was a former Laker's Cheer Leader - it took all my strength, endurance and determination to stay the course. But, I did it!

Shortly afterwards, I had both my hips replaced at the same time! During my long recovery, my husband and I designed and constructed a yoga studio in our backyard. Then, I began to invite people to train with me and began building a fulfilling new career.

I am now 82 years old and feel better physically, emotionally and spiritually than I have since my 50s. My husband plays music at the end of my classes and also takes my Chair Yoga sessions three times a week.

It gives us a shared activity, purpose and responsibility - which keeps us happy, healthy and connected to a community which we have formed.

These past 12 years - since I wrote my revised Long Range Plan - have brought a youthful exuberance to our lives, and connected us to a diverse group of people who share the joy of being healthy together. Although we may have a variety of differing interests, philosophies and political bents, we find that age does not interfere in our ability to connect as members of the human family. We not only practice yoga together, but we support each other in fulfilling our lives.

My motto is quite simple: *"Never give up!"*

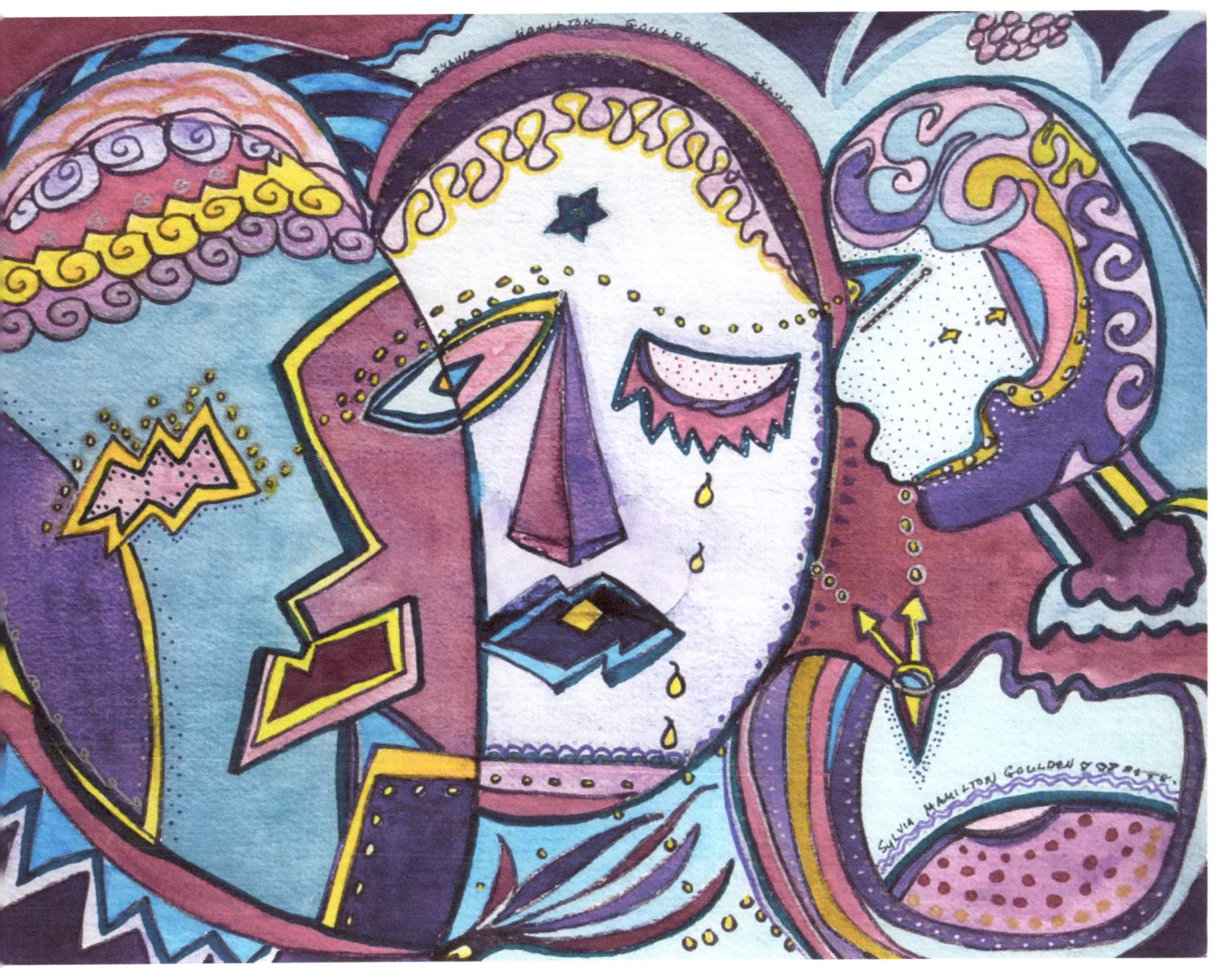

#2 What are the Masks and Costumes You Love to Wear?

Why do so many people love costumes and masks? On Halloween or during Mardi Gras, people feel they've been given permission to take on different personas. But, what about in their everyday lives? Perhaps we sometimes hide behind a mask we have fashioned for our natural face – a smile, a frown, a blank stare, a look that will frighten, or an expression that shows we don't care (even when we really do).

From earliest times, people told stories around an evening fire – mysterious tales of the hunt, of great danger and bravery, or the adventures of a journey. They added masks to their stories, animal skins and disguises to increase the impact for their audiences.

It's interesting that even though we have different beliefs and customs, the foundational elements for all humans have little variation. Our stories feature similar archetypes, differing only in the variety of body structures, colors, sizes, textures and personalities. According to the Swiss psychiatrist, Carl Jung (1875-1961), there are various types of people. Writer, Kendra Cherry, explains; *"Archetypes are universal, inborn models of people, behaviors, or personalities that play a role in influencing human behavior."*

Here are just a few archetypes from Carl Jung:

- **The father:** authority figure; stern; powerful
- **The mother:** nurturing; comforting
- **The child:** longing for innocence; rebirth; salvation
- **The wise old man:** guidance; knowledge; wisdom
- **The hero:** champion; defender; rescuer
- **The maiden:** innocen ce, desire; purity
- **The trickster:** deceiver; liar; trouble-maker

The mythic characters that represent these archetypes are found world-wide, and in all cultures. Each of us leans toward one or more of these types, determined by such things as culture, religion, dreams, art or personality. As children, we learn what to do and how to behave in order to fit into the world. Thus, we often create "masks" to wear as we interact with others.

The mythic character s that represent these archetypes are found world-wide, and in all cultures. Each of us leans toward one or more of these types, determined by such things as culture, religion, dreams, art or personality.

As children, we learn what to do and how to behave in order to fit into the world. Thus, we often create "masks" to wear as we interact with others.

Jung divided them into four major archetypal groups. The first is The Persona, which in Latin means "mask." It is the way in which we present ourselves to the world. The others are, *The Shadow, The Anima or Animus,* and *The Self.* I will focus on *The Persona* and *The Self.*

When we are young, we make certain decisions about ourselves, partially because of our innate personalities - and partially because of the order of our birth and circumstances. We learn how to role-play early on as we study people to see how to get what we want. There are also people whom we admire or fear, and we often choose to take on traits of people who seem to have the most power. We mask our face and body, acting this character out in life as a substitute for our *True Self.* We try on the trickster, heroine, father or mother.

What archetype are you? What role do you like to play? Are you this persona when you are alone? What mask do you wear to family gatherings? To work? Who are you when you spend time with friends? How is your persona different from the person you secretly know yourself to be? Think about it!

But, of course, the most important question is, *"Who are you without your persona?"* That is the challenge in *Living Your Now.*

#3 What is Loving Kindness?

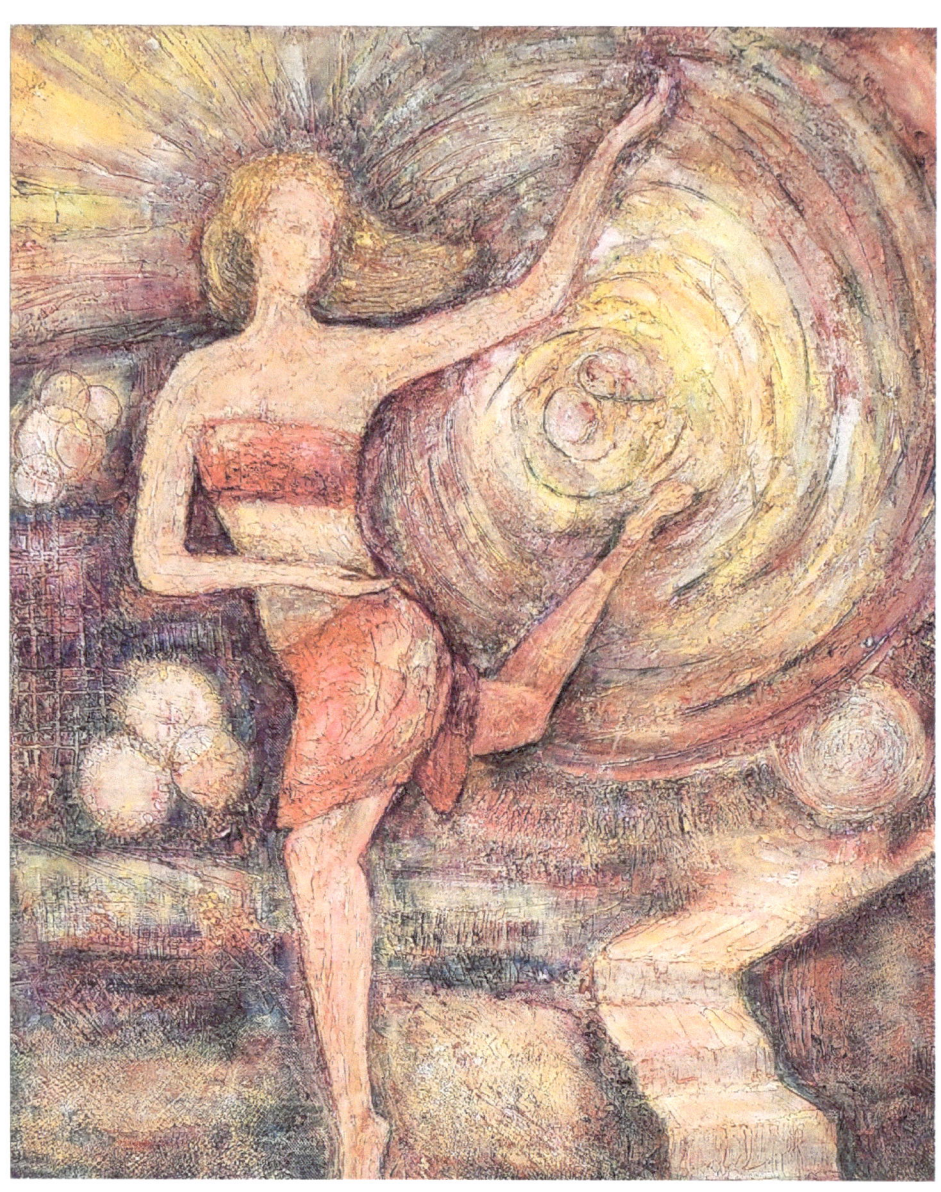

Loving – a person who is capable of generating and flowing kind energy to themselves and others.

Kindness – the quality of being friendly, generous, respectful, and considerate.

Here is an anonymous poem, based on ancient wisdom, that simply and powerfully shows the impact of our actions on others.

KINDNESS

Drop a stone into the water –
In a moment it is gone,
But there are a hundred ripples
circling on and on and on.

Say an unkind word this moment –
In a moment it is gone,
But there are a hundred ripples
circling on and on and on.

Say a word of cheer and splendor –
In a moment it is gone,
But there are a hundred ripples
circling on and on and on.

When we say something unkind, or even mean, we don't always know the impact it has on people. Lifelong scars may be formed by these people to protect themselves, causing them to feel shame, expect less, or even take on the very behavior that was so destructive to them

In the same way, we don't always know that our kind and loving gestures or words will lift someone up.

One of the strategies we use to protect ourselves is to think less of who we are. Some people develop a lifetime of sadness or anger - even rage. Others simple feel worthless, not believing that they deserve a good partner, career, work situation, or personal happiness.

The current Dalai Lama says, *"My religion is kindness."* I really like this! It's simple and straight to the point of what really makes us feel noticed, valued and accepted. I can easily think back on moments throughout my life when I was sad, felt worthless and unseen. Then, a kind person gave me a smile and an encouraging word - and, immediately I felt uplifted. It's truly amazing how a person of any gender, race or age, with a quick, generous word can break through the walls we build to protect ourselves.

Of course, this is often a role that our pets play in our lives, as they look at us with expectant joy, curiosity or interest. They easily rub themselves against our legs, climb up into our laps, give us a purr, cuddle or an enthusiastic jump! Sometimes they just lie down beside us - or on top of us - and fall asleep in that most accepting of ways.

How do we become more loving and kind? Is this even possible?

Yes, I believe that it is possible to become more loving and kind. But it all needs to begin within. Before we can truly feel worthy of someone else's love and appreciation, we need to begin by accepting and loving ourselves. We can decide to close our eyes and connect to our own hearts. This is where loving kindness resides - although sometimes it has been held prisoner. Some of us have tightened the muscles around our heart, preventing us from feeling safe - relaxing into love, kindness, compassion, acceptance and inclusion. A saddened, fearful, or angry heart, can isolate us from others, building a wall against attacks or shame.

So, here is something you might like to try, to free your own heart from your sadness, fear and anger:

1. Sit or lie comfortably in a quiet indoor or outdoor space.

2. Gently close your eyes; take a few moments to breathe deeply.

3. Imagine a place of beauty; place yourself in the middle of this scene.

4. Decide it is safe to open your heart a tiny bit and receive the energy of the beauty that surrounds you.

5. Breathe in and let the energy flow into your heart - feel the effects.

6. Then, on your exhales, let the locked up love in your heart release and flow outwards.

7. Repeat this several times - feel the ease and confidence that begins.

Being loving and kind begins with oneself. It is the way we nourish ourselves with positive energy. Eventually, you become a reservoir of loving kindness and radiate it out to everyone you contact!

#4 How Do I Flow Loving Kindness When I Don't Feel Loving?

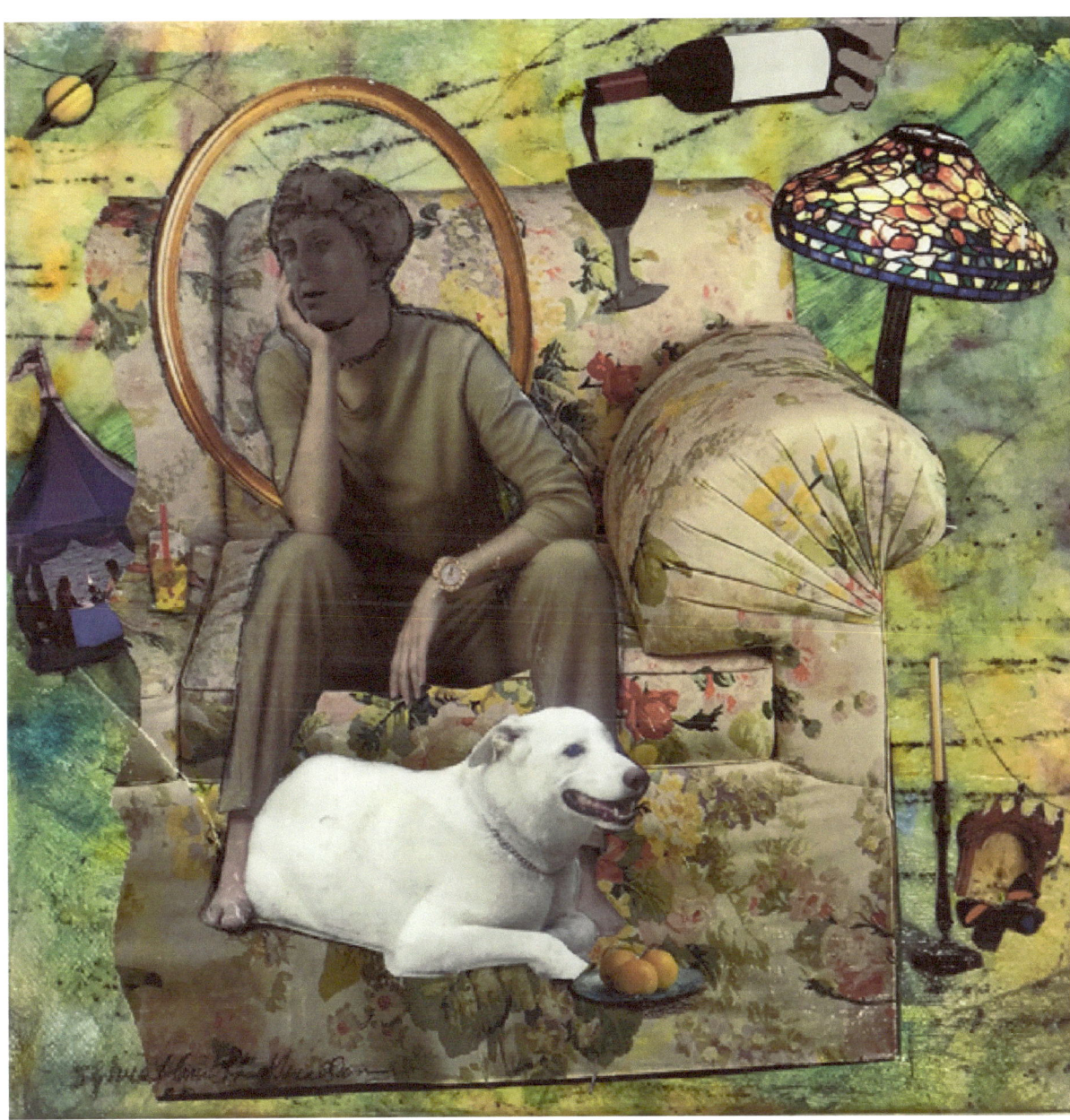

All of us – if we are honest – have felt unloving at times. This is normal. Perhaps we are depressed, lonely or have suffered a big letdown. From my experience, it begins with me not loving myself, or feeling unworthy of love and kindness. When this happens, I unconsciously invite people to withdraw, shut me out, or use me as their own punching bag. I react by being sullen, fearful or angry. I am not being loved by others, so why should I flow love out into this hostile, uncaring world? This is a natural response – but it is not helpful or productive to becoming happy.

Happiness starts deep within ourselves.

"Happiness will never come to those who fail to appreciate what they already have."

Bilal Zahoor

I have found that I can begin to change my inner atmosphere from negative to positive by beginning with gratitude. I start each morning in my bath. Lying back in piles of soft bubbles, I start at my toes and move up my torso, giving thanks to each body part that serves me. I overlook my flaws and focus on what is good. I thank each part for serving me so well – every day! It's amazing how this shifts my focus from what I am lacking to how many parts of me are working well. It is rather a miracle! Our bodies are complex and yet completely synchronized.

Our breath, for example, can operate automatically, or be controlled by our mind – and, our breath affects our emotional state, focus and well-being.

Begin by consciously releasing your heart to flow kindness and love to yourself.

I teach my yoga students to begin with breathing. A good beginning for this is to inhale for 4 counts; pause; exhale for 4 counts; pause. Breathing in and out through the nose, do this pattern 8 cycles. Notice how you feel afterwards. Then, bring both palms together at your sternum (breast bone). Continuing to take deep, smooth breaths, think of three things that you can be grateful for. These can be events, things, people, the environment or having food, water and clean air.

Feeling gratitude frees the muscles around your heart. The closed "doors" of your heart begin to open and love flows unfettered. First, let these positive sensations touch every cell of your body. These are healing forces. This positive energy expands quickly when given permission to do so. Give it permission!

This can be followed by the Loving Kindness Meditation which has four basic steps:

1. Flow love and kindness to oneself.

2. Think of someone you love and flow love and kindness to that person.

3. Think of a stranger – someone you have seen, but don't know – and flow love and kindness to them

4. Think of someone who you find difficult, don't like, are angry with, or have been hurt by. This is the hardest of all – but flow loving kindness to them. While it is challenging, it is also freeing. It is your own heart that will heal and expand.

Finally, I have an affirmation that I say daily:

I am enough.

Yes, you are enough just the way you are. You are unique. Even if you are a twin, there is only one of you. Life has a beginning, middle and an end. Do not waste the middle part being sad, isolated, fearful or angry. Here is a favorite quote by Abraham Lincoln:

"We can complain because rose bushes have thorns,
Or rejoice because thorn bushes have roses."

Each life is full of suffering and each life has the capacity for joy, connection and fulfillment. The antidote for suffering is loving kindness toward yourself and all others.

#5 Embracing Change in Our Lives

The core of Patanjali's *Yoga Sutra* is an eight-limbed path that forms the structural framework for yoga practice. In this essay I will explore the first four limbs: the *Yamas* (universal truths), Niamas (personal truths), *Asanas* (poses) and *Pranayama* (breath or life force). The main focus will be on how to embrace change in the process of aging with an emphasis on Santosa (contentment with what we have) and Syadhyaya (self-study).

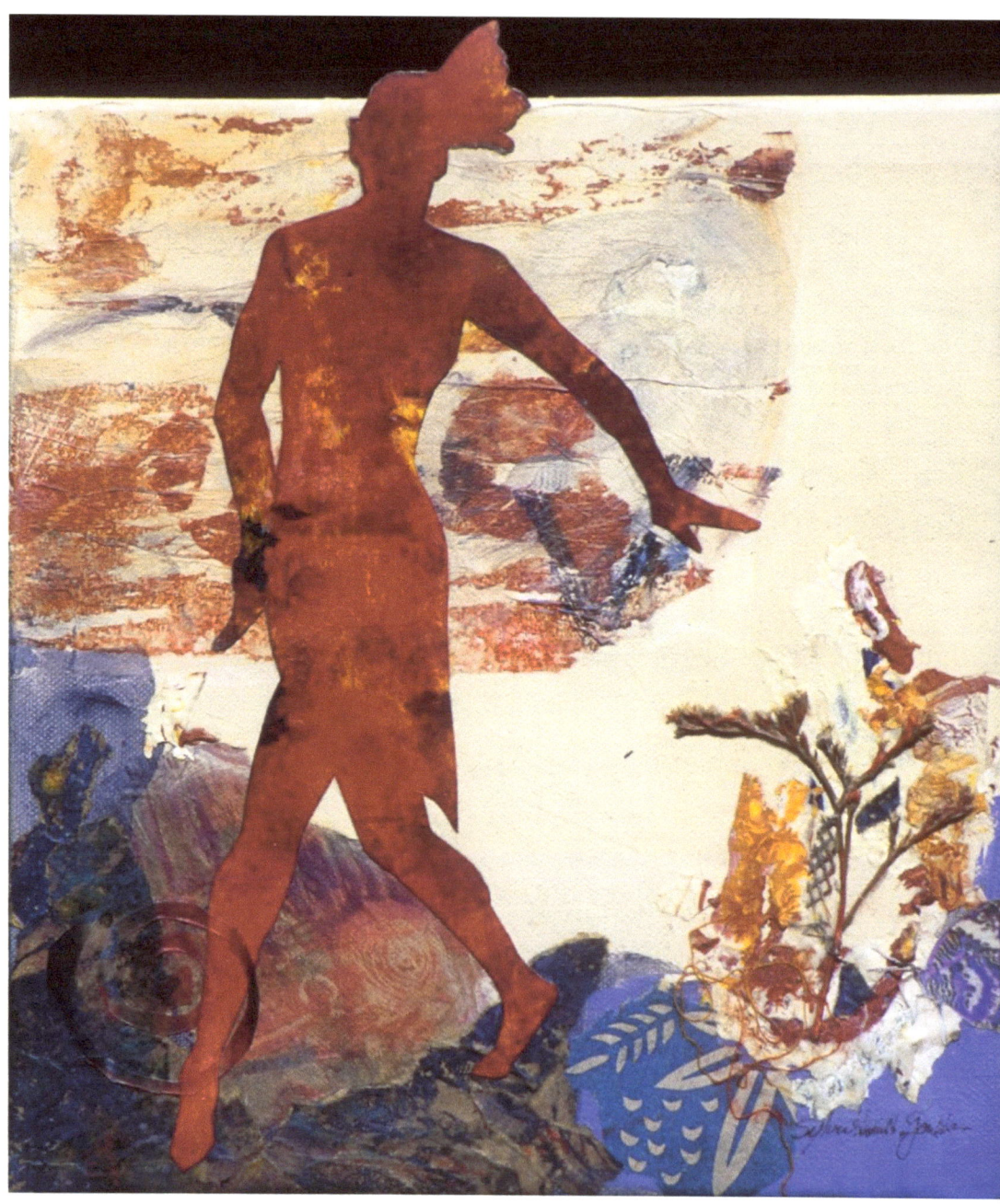

"To be content doesn't mean you don't desire more, it means you're thankful for what you have and patient for what's to come."
Tony Gaskins

This commentary on the Sutras is found in the book, In the Heart of Yoga: Developing a Personal Practice, by TK.V Desikachar.

In investigating the essence of Santosa, you are encouraged to contemplate your attitudes about growing older. To embark upon a journey of self discovery and self appreciation, you will need to deal with change. How comfortable are you with change? Do you resist making changes in your life - or work to keep things as they have always been?

Can you allow yourself to consider the chosen and non-chosen changes in your life without self judgment and doubt?

With increased awareness, we can work toward changing our attitude in our thoughts and in the physical practice of yoga.

As changes are made, it's helpful to have attitudes such as curiosity, inquiry, discovery and responsibility to oneself

Here is an excerpt from The Desiderata, a poem by Max Ehrmann.

"Take kindly the counsel of the years, gracefully surrendering the things of youth.

*You are a child of the universe
no less than the trees and the stars.
You have a right to be here.
And whether or not it is clear to you,
no doubt the universe is unfolding as it should.*

Come, join me on this "Journey of Discovery" and claim a new and positive attitude about getting older and changing. The best is still to come, even though we may not be able to see around the next corner.

#6 My Own Journey Through Change

I have lived through more than seven decades of this confusing adventure called "life." I know from personal experience that yoga practice, beyond the poses, has the potential to help you find increased freedom by fully embracing who you truly are. As I have aged, I have come closer to understanding a small corner of this concept of living more fully in each moment. This came about through focused self-study, yoga classes and workshops. A more positive attitude has led me to a deeper acceptance and contentment in all aspects of my life. I have also gained a deeper level of gratitude for all I have been given and continue to receive.

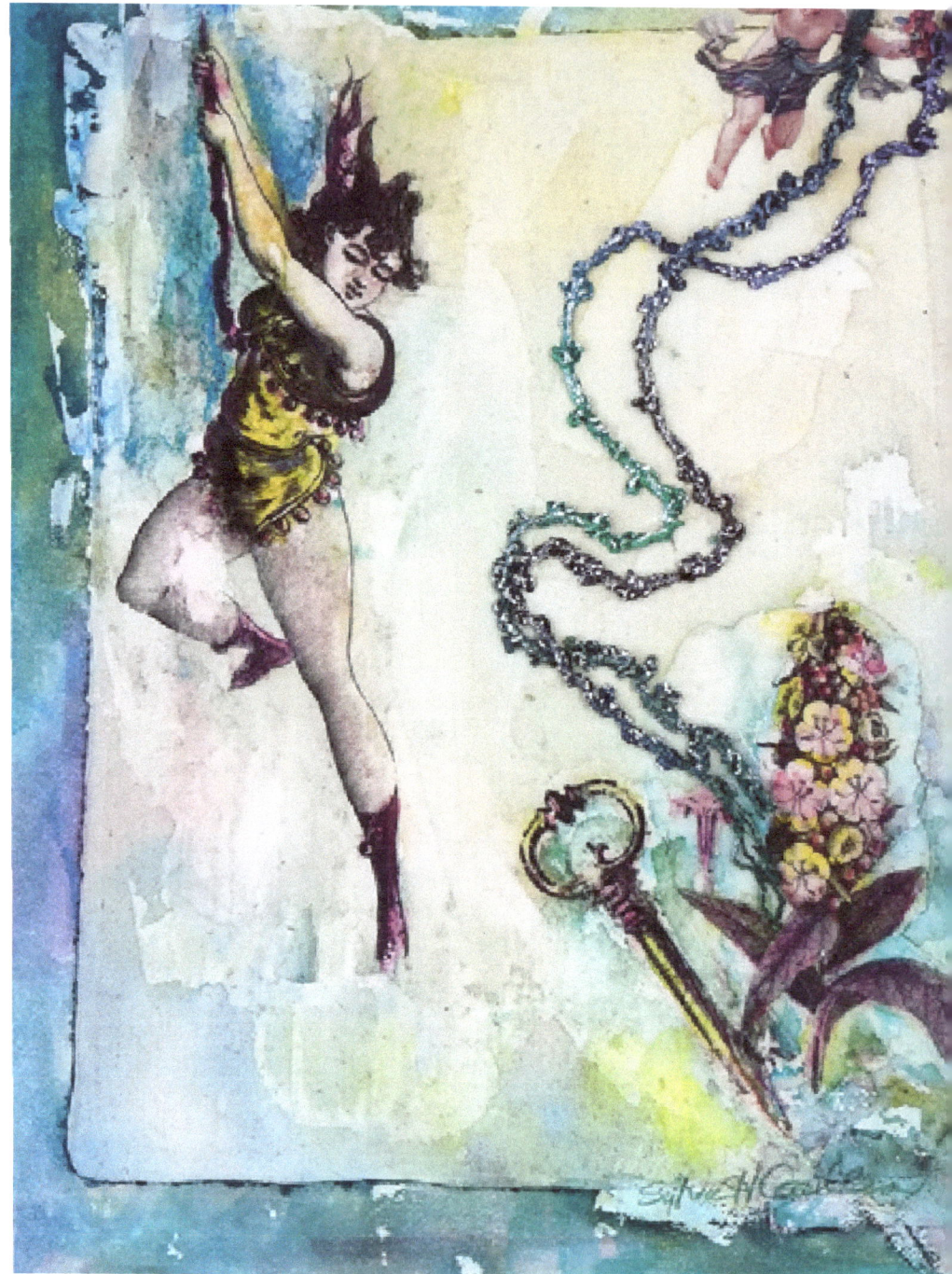

My study of the Yoga Sutras have connected me more fully with the Yamas and the Niyamas, (*"The Yamas and the Niyamas"* by Deborah Adele) and I have been inspired to write my "Personal Code of Honor" which I strive to fulfill. These universal and personal ideals have helped me find deeper meaning in my own purpose. I have made progress toward accepting what is, and lessened my need to control people or outcomes. For me the concept of Santosa began with the feeling that I can trust in the process of my life as it unfolds. Earlier, several tragic experiences brought me to my knees. I came to a point where I had to make a decision whether to be in constant pain for the rest of my life, or change. I finally surrendered to my pain and let it engulf me. In my suffering I received many gifts of insight tucked into its dark pockets. With very small steps in the beginning, I eventually began to free my spirit by forgiving myself and others, and dealing with change. I realized that everyone I knew, especially close friends and family, needed me to heal.

I now envision myself as a lighthouse, guiding others as they navigate their way through life. After more than 25 years of practice, I became a yoga teacher at age 70. I wanted to share the knowledge and tools that enabled me to embrace change and the process of growth - which is optional.

Wherever you are in your life, change is the only constant. But, there is hope! Yoga offers us ancient wisdom and strategies to be more present, to release negative energy, and to fuel our vitality.

Because we are all part of this human experience, these principles are as valid today as they were 5,000 years ago!

#7 Forgiveness

The first thing to remember is that when you forgive someone, you are doing it for yourself It allows you to move on from a painful experience, and release yourself from being negatively bound to another.

Here is a great quote that helps you remember the destructive energy of resentment and anger, and the healing balm of release from negative emotions.

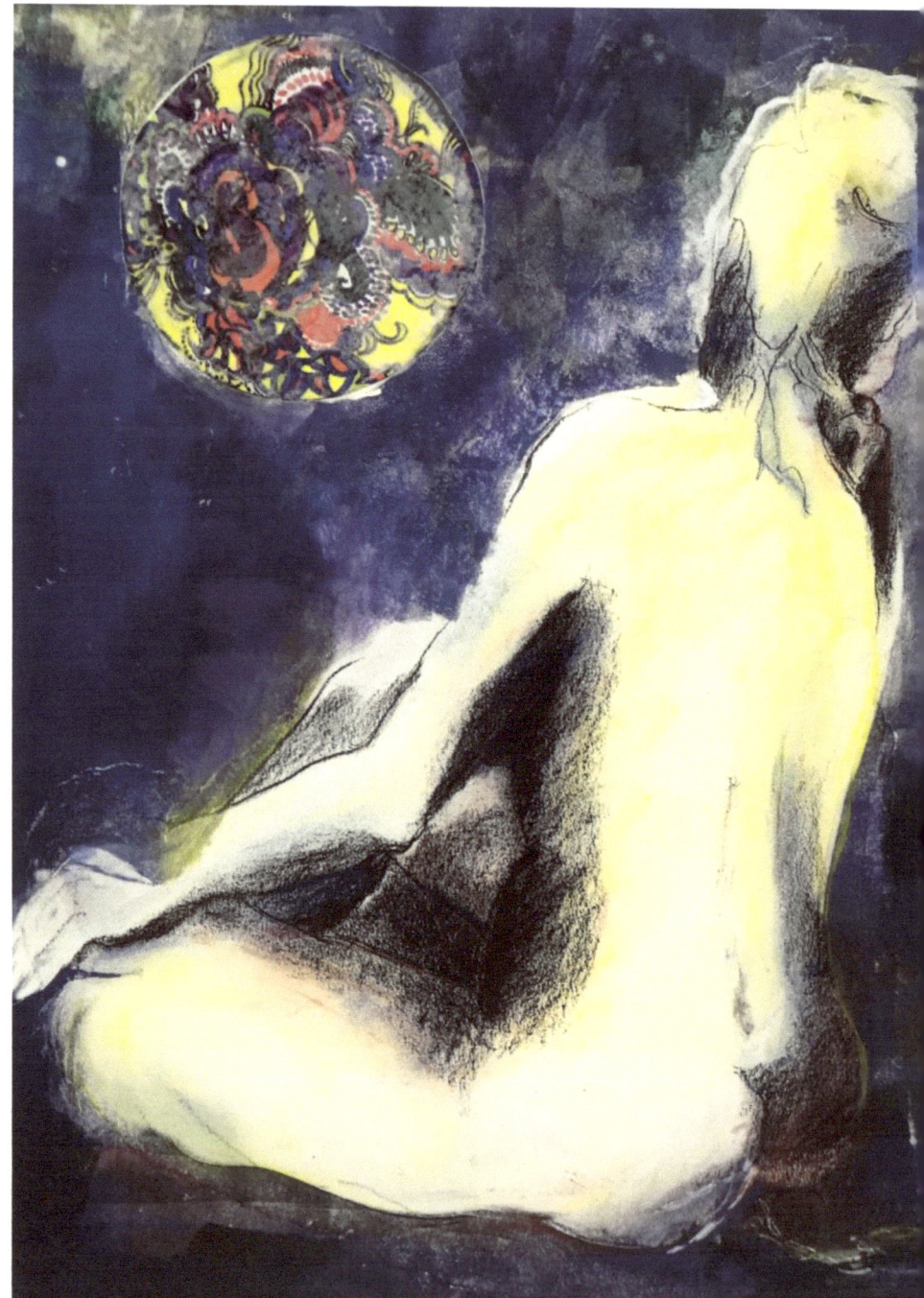

Forgiveness doesn't
Excuse their behavior
Forgiveness prevents
Their behavior from
Destroying your heart.

Beyond Ordinary

This poem inspired me to write my own.

Why I Forgive You

I feel hurt, wounded.
Your words explode like bullets,
    causing hemorrhage
    and pain within my soul.
How did I become your target?
Why do you wish to hurt,
    belittle and shame me?
I don't know what I've done
    to hurt you so.
Do I remind you of someone
    who pierced you with pain?
Perhaps someone in your past,
    someone close to you.
Is that why you push me away?
Is this why you set me up
    for failure and ridicule?

Does this make you feel strong?
Do you weaken me to find courage?

I reach out in friendship.
You respond by throwing mud –
    blurring my vision,
    disorienting me,
    lessening my value,
    covering me with your
    soiled emotions.

I don't like what you do.
I don't like the way you
    make me feel.
I don't want you in my life.
I don't want the tainted
    gifts you bear.

Instead, I forgive you.
What you have done is unkind.
But, it's more about you than me.
I am kind and generous.
You are troubled and cruel.

Yet, I forgive you because
    it frees me, not you.

Susan Cambigue Tracey

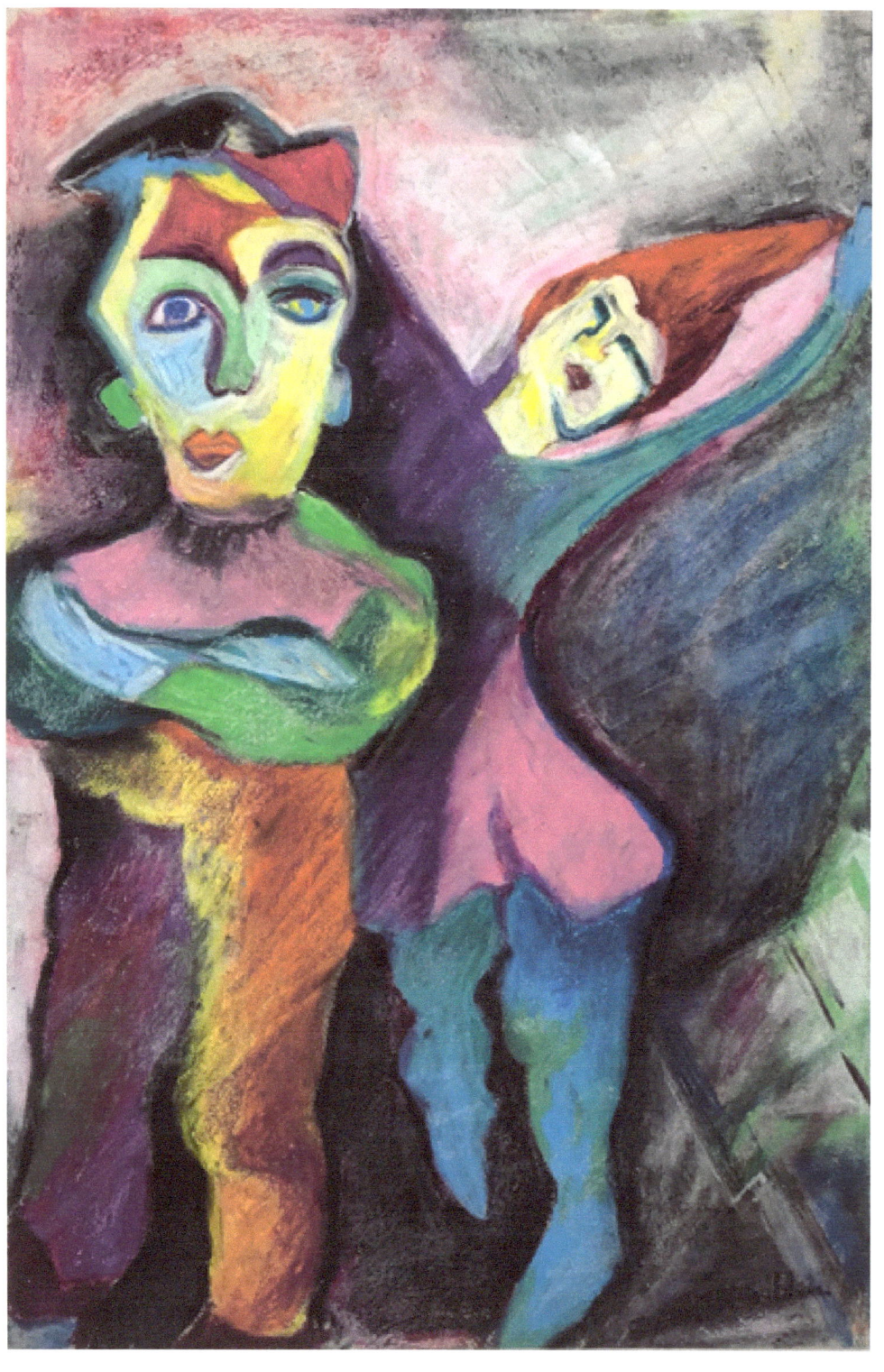

#8 Revisiting Br'er Rabbit and The Tar Baby

A sticky, ickey, gooey mess!
The intriguing Tar Baby,
a doll made of
tar and turpentine.
Br'er Rabbit trapped in black, thick goo
difficult to extricate himself.

African American tale
rooted in the iniquities of slavery.
Some people have control –
others are under their control.

Br'er Rabbit - a trickster -
is entrapped by
the villainous Br'er Fox.
Fox wants to inflict maximum pain!
He now controls the rabbit -
but, the rabbit plays the wise victim,
freeing himself with a suggestion
that Fox throw him in the Briar Patch!

Fox is evil and punishing -
so he does just that!
And–
Br'er Rabbit escapes - it is his home!

Tar Baby is a metaphor for
a sticky situation that gets worse
the more one struggles.
Stop fighting the injustice
inflicted by another.
Release yourself from their
gooey, tangled trap.
Think, rather than react!

Free yourself from
this glutinous drama.
Discover release from
playing the victim's role
in someone else's play. Don't
accept the part
they force upon you.
Don't get enmeshed in
someone else's pain.
Hot, gummy words and
actions trap you.
The more you struggle, the
more anger and sorrow
adheres to your skin -
keeping you wrapped
in dark, persistent emotions.
Sit in the light.
Let the tacky mess melt,
dripping onto the earth,
absorbed and transformed, it
has no more power over
you.

Susan Cambigue Tracey

Historical note: Br'er Rabbit is a trickster figure originating in Africa, and transmitted by slaves to the new world, in the form of stories

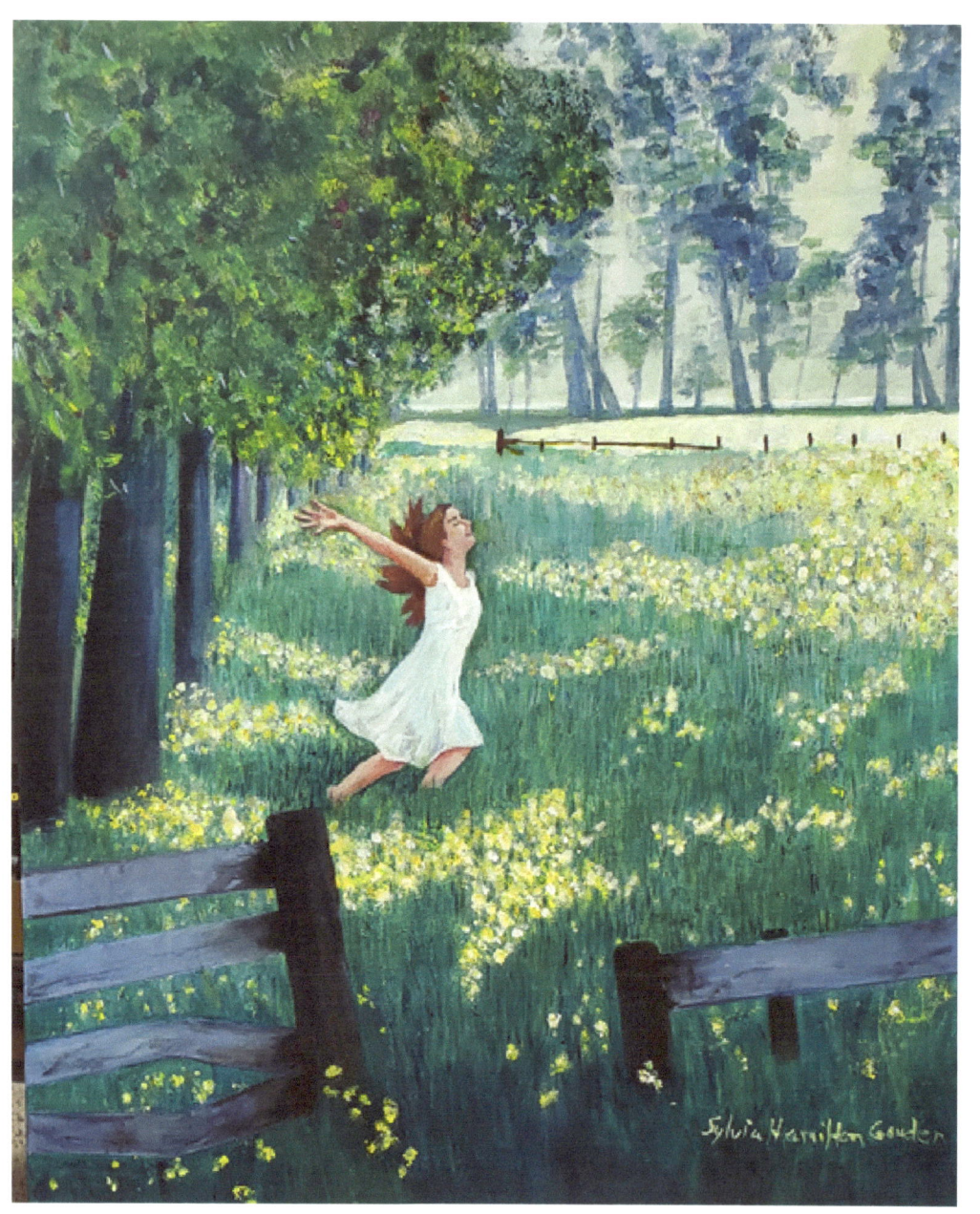

#9 New Beginnings - An Empowering Meditation

January 1st is my favorite day of the year! Better than New Year's Eve, it represents the possibilities of new beginnings. Here is a meditation from a woman named Jaspa, who taught at Crossroads Elementary School in Santa Monica.

The ideas are what I remember from a faculty meditation she guided more than 30 years ago. The elaboration on these concepts are my own.

Here is my script to guide you. I suggest you consider making a simple recording of yourself reading the following meditation. If you want to elaborate, add some non-vocal music with guitar, flute, strings, singing bowls or other soft, yet inspiring sounds.

TREE AND BLOSSOM MEDITATION

Begin with breath - Inhale for 4 counts; Pause; Exhale for 4 counts; Pause. (Repeat 4 - 8 times)

"Imagine yourself as a tree of your choice.

Put down strong roots into the earth.

Spread out your branches and place buds, blossoms and blooms on the branches. Make them any colors you like.

Now let your spirit float around and through your tree, and see it clearly.

Notice that some of the flowers are just buds, some are beginning to open and others are fully in bloom.

Float over to one of the flowers that is fully open and look inside to see which of your talents or gifts you are using fully. What trait or quality have you allowed to blossom within yourself?

Now, acknowledge that gift and then move on to another full blossom. What do you see within? What gift are you realizing? Acknowledge it.

Breath in deeply and feel the fulfillment in using these gifts, and the joy and satisfaction it brings you.

Now, travel over to a bud that is just beginning to blossom - to open up. What do you see within its petals? What within you is ready to be realized, ready to bloom? What needs a bit more encouragement? Can you allow this blossom to fully open? Can you accept its gift?

Now, float over to the tightly bound buds on the tree. Select one to study. What do you see inside? What is its potential? Are you willing to give it the permission and energy to open and be seen?

Finally, what are you willing to let go of? What blossoms are ready to be released to fall away? What have you finished with? What has had its moment, and is now over?

Ending: breathe deeply, with an intensified sense of understanding, of acceptance and compassion for yourself, your dreams and your disappointments. Feel yourself as the tree, with the potential to grow and continue to flower."

#10 Self Study- Trust Your Own Process

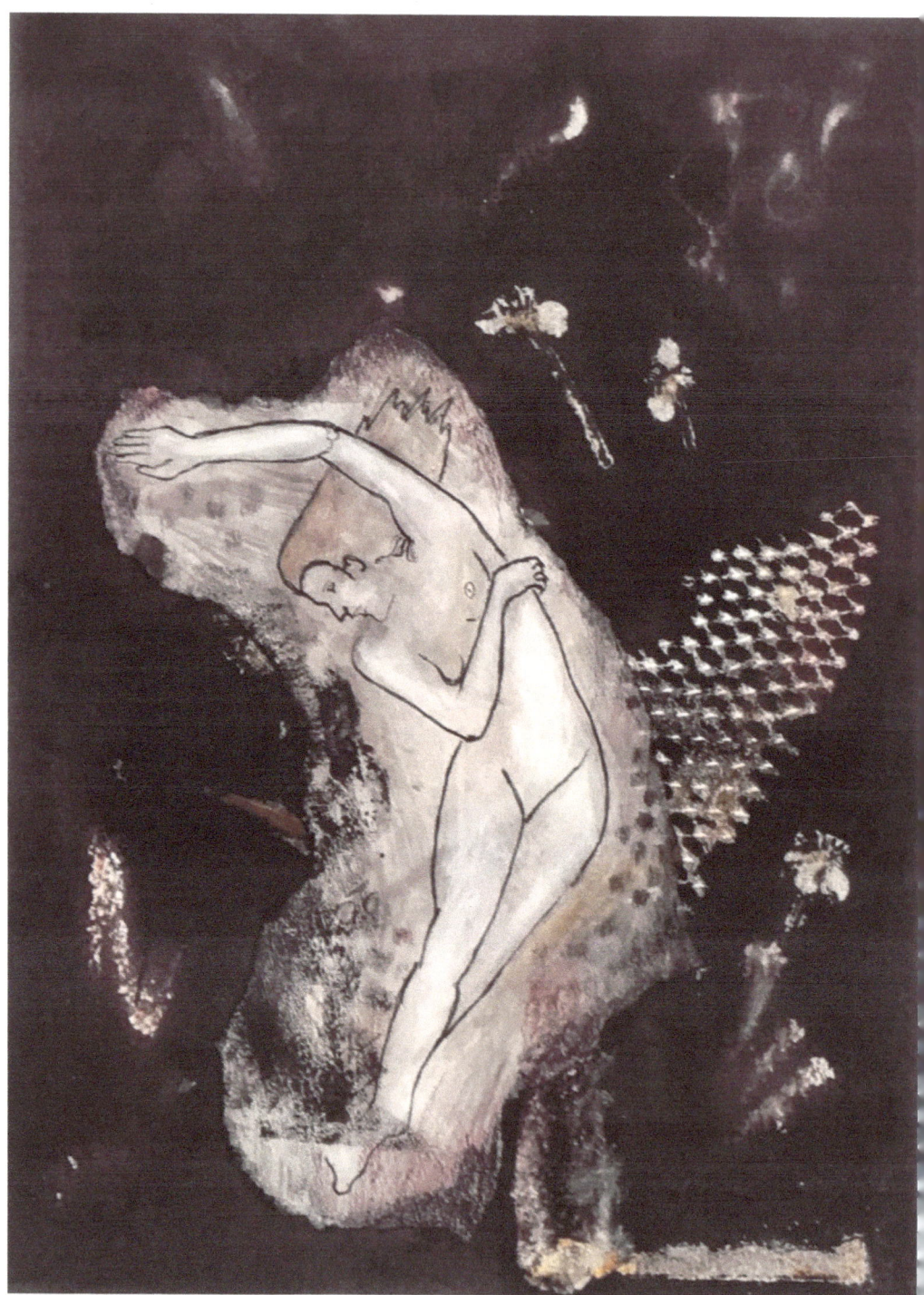

Svadhyaya is a Sanskrit term for Indian traditions that promote positive values for living a meaningful life. It is based on the virtue of self-study and is a system for self-transformation. Part of the *Niyamas,* on the second limb of the yoga tree, this category of concepts serve as principles ideally observed and practiced. These rules are about developing optimum human traits and habits.

It involves the study of spiritual texts and introspection - looking within oneself for answers. The main emphasis in self-study is finding a path to follow that leads one to have enlightened moments of thought.

Self-study, the fourth of the five niyamas - or personal observances - is about getting out of your own way. To help people cease stumbling over unnoticed pebbles or going round and round the hamster's wheel, self study makes one more aware and responsible.

We may feel exhausted with the effort we expend to move forward, but nothing changes. You are basically stuck. Something within you needs to wake up; realize that some attitude must alter for true change to occur.

One of my students at Loyola Marymount University in Los Angeles was taking a required course from me. She made it clear that she found little value in the course, which centered on dance education. However, she changed during the semester, and by winter break she was deeply engaged. When she finished the course, she gave me a small gift - it was a magnet she made with this saying:

*"Nothing has changed except my attitude;
Therefore, everything has changed."*

That truth stayed on my refrigerator for ten years, when it finally lost its magnetism, but not the power of its words. That's OK because I got the teaching.

Once we let down our defenses and remain naked in our aloneness, we actually become more comfortable in our skin.

I love self study, and write my musings on a regular basis. It helps me to express my feelings and to gain more clarity about what is actually at the center of my malaise. Why do the same upsets occur over and over? Why do we continue to attract people with similar attributes – personalities and traits that press our emotional red buttons? Think about it!

I continue to follow the advice of author Julia Cameron, who wrote the classic book, *The Artist's Way*. She advised us to write "Morning Pages" everyday and to use them as a way to clear the clutter out of our mind. It wasn't to write something publishable, but rather to empty our minds to think more clearly.

I remember having absolutely nothing to write one day, so I just started observing everything in my kitchen that was white. I was surprised to find items I hadn't noticed in a while. After some time, it became more of a lighthearted game. I was intrigued, and for about an hour, I developed a piece on whiteness, working each line to be more poetic. I became enthused and filled with new possibilities.

WHITE

Sitting in my sun-filled kitchen,
I am suddenly aware of
    the white paint on the walls,
    sunbeams bouncing off them
    into the room.
White surrounds me,
    also above me on the ceiling!
White daisies pose in a
    blue vase on the table.
A white fridge holds my food
the white stove stands
    ready to cook it.
A white bowl of cereal
    sits before me,
    sprinkled with white sugar,
    covered in a sea of white milk.
I dip my spoon into
    the white waves of liquid,
    grinding the flakes
    with my rows of white teeth.
My eyes, embedded in a white background,
    watch that I don't spill.
Pulling my white sweater more
    tightly around my shoulders,
I feel cozy in my colorless world.

I wrote Morning Pages for a full year – gaining new vision and insight into myself. Julia recommends that one doesn't read what has been written for several weeks or months. When I did sit down to read my collection of daily writings, I was surprised at how my clearest thoughts came through faster and my complaints decreased.

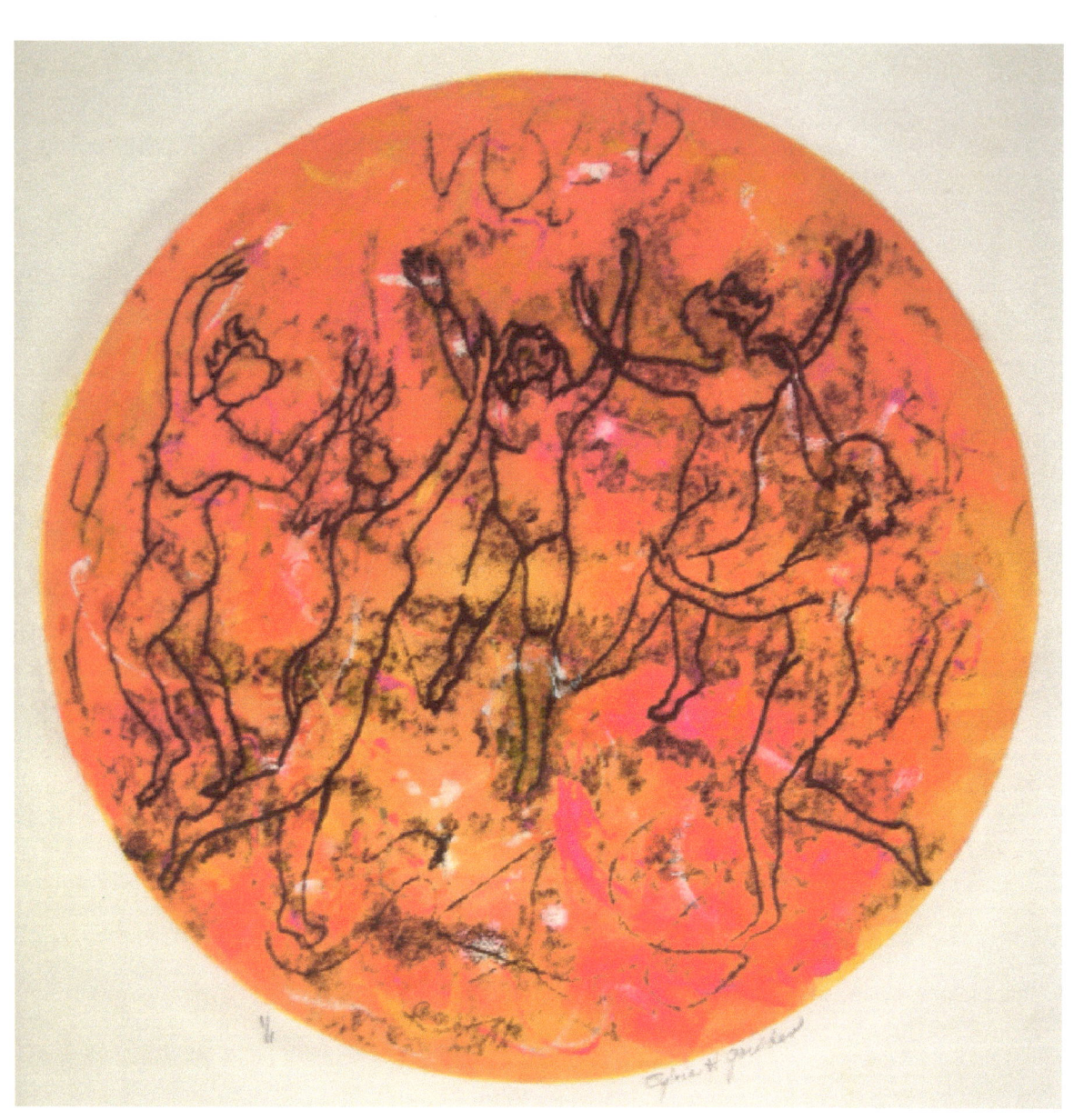

#11 How I Authentically Connect with Others

As a child I wondered, as all children do, what my future would hold. Until I was twelve, I spent countless hours playing with my dolls, setting up different situations so I could practice real life relationships.

Every night it was agony to decide which of them would sleep with me. This long ritual became longer still when I included all of them in my prayers, along with my family and friends.

I remember one particular night. My mother was putting me to bed when it suddenly dawned on me – people are the most important thing in life!

With this revelation, I transferred my attention from dolls to people – building a wide variety of friendships . My truest friends have always been honest, loving and supportive. They have enabled me to uncover, and discover, my true self. What a gift friendship offers!

Most of my friends are women who have courageously faced many challenges. They have given deeply and freely of their gifts. Inspired and guided by others, they have developed their own characters by the choices they have made. Most did not take an easy route, but rather a challenging one. Struggles were faced, not pushed aside for an easier life.

Yet, in spite of the struggles they each faced, they found strength and support from enduring friendships.

These friendships began with shared values – honesty and fairness, kindness and sincerity, a connection to curiosity, creativity, and being keen observers .

My particular friends all have an urge to stand up for such ideals as inclusion, loving kindness and acceptance of ourselves and others, and opportunities, liberty and justice for all. We show up for each other, we listen to each other, we celebrate each other's successes, and comfort each other when we experience loss.

To sum it up, I am attracted to friends who see the things they have, rather than what they are missing. Whether shy or outgoing, they each have a "joie de vivre" – a joyful enthusiasm for the possibilities in life. To arrive at this clarity, it is necessary to let go of ideas like trying to impress, wearing personas rather than being authentic, gossiping about others' flaws and bsses .

The painting by Sylvia Hamilton Goulden that accompanies this essay is called "Dance as One." Here is a haiku which she wrote to embellish it.

"Dancing as one mind
Friends through the season of life
Gather their power."

Here are a few wise quotes about friendship that I find valuable:

"The most beautiful discovery true friends make is that they can grow separately without growing apart."
　　　　　　　　　　　　Elizabeth Foley

"If ever there is a tomorrow when we're not together… there is something you must always remember. You are braver than you believe, stronger than you seem, and smarter than you think but the most important thing is, even if we're apart…
I'll always be with you."
　　　　　　　　　　　　Winnie the Pooh
　　　　　　　　　　　　Attributed to A.A. Milne

"Good friends help you to find important things when you have lost them… your smile, your hope, and your courage."
　　　　　　　　　　　　Doe Zantamata

"Don't walk behind me; I may not lead.
Don't walk in front of me; I may not follow.
Just walk beside me and be my friend."
　　　　　　　　　　　　Albert Camus

#12 Taking Responsibility for the Health of our Planet.
Essay by Paul Tracey

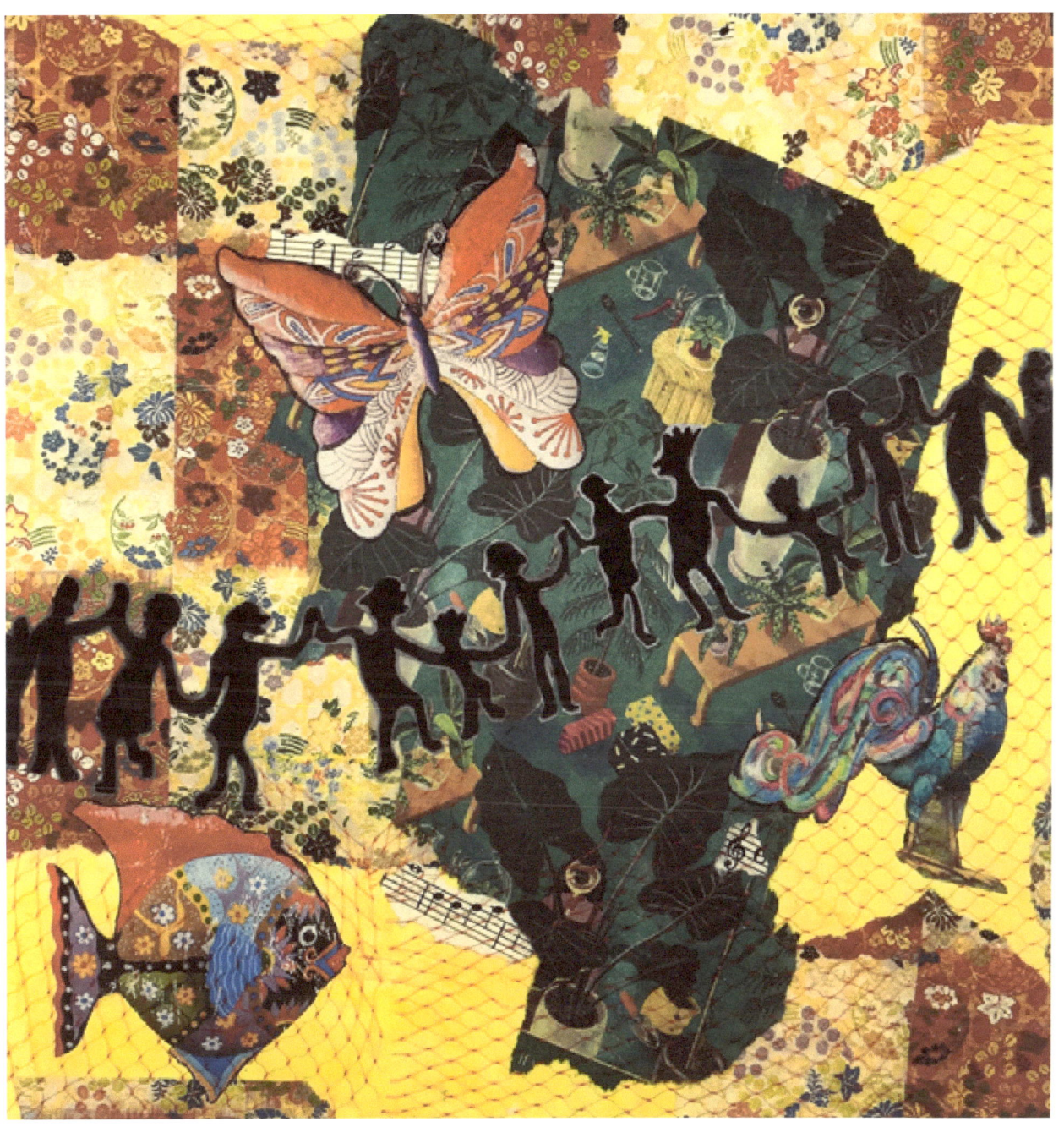

"Our Little Blue Planet, Our home out in space;
Without your environment, No human race;
No fish in the ocean, No birds in no trees,
No monkeys in forests,
No dogs with no fleas. (yowl!)"

For almost 50 years I gave myself the job of creating and performing entertaining and educational performances for school audiences. The challenge I faced in 1988 was this: how could I create *Our Little Blue Planet* - a 45 minute assembly program for elementary school children that could inspire them to treat our planet with the respect and love it deserves, all without sounding preachy?

I grew up on a farm in England's West Country in the County of Somerset- the locals pronounce it "Zomerzet." We had an orchard of cider apples there, "zider" they said, which was sold to make "scrumpy" which is the local version of hard cider.

So naturally I was raised being very much aware of nature and how farmers relate to it, preserving it for the future so its products could always be sold to the public to keep us all alive.

City dwellers didn't have the same advantages that I had, so I knew that my environmental assembly could play an important role in educating city kids in these times of global warming and climate change, when preservation of all things natural is becoming more and more critical.

Perhaps more important even than food production, is access to breathable air. Oxygen is a vital element, but where do we find it? One major source comes from trees and their ability to photosynthesize, using sunlight. I know about trees. I practically grew up in one - a beech tree where I had a hammock way up, three stories high. Little did I know then how important those lovely, light green leaves were to our very existence.